PRAISE FOR
DR. ELENA ZINKOV, ND

For many of us, the challenge is not how to choose the best foods, it is about how to follow through with our best choices. By in large, diets are sabotaged by cravings, not food errors. In *Crave Reset*, Dr. Zinkov will guide you through a plan to help the best-documented triggers of cravings so that you can live life to your best intentions and regain ideal health.

—Alan Christianson, NMD
NY Times Bestselling author of *The Adrenal Reset Diet*

"At the root of food cravings is a primal impulse that drives us toward pleasure. In Crave Reset, Dr. Zinkov combines the science of cravings with hands-on solutions to help people achieve peak health regardless of their genetic predisposition."

—Robb Wolf, New York Times bestselling author of
The Paleo Solution and *Wired to Eat, The Paleo Solution Podcast*

"Dr. Elena Zinkov has put together a whole-self, complete guide to understanding cravings, allowing the reader to mine their deep messages for body and mind. When we heal our relationship with food, we open up to our inner spectrum of potential in new ways that allow us to feel empowered and energized."

— Deanna Minich, PhD, health expert and author, *Whole Detox*

CRAVE
RESET

A BREAKTHROUGH GUIDE *for* MASTERING *the* PSYCHOLOGY *and* PHYSIOLOGY *of* CRAVINGS

DR. ELENA ZINKOV ND

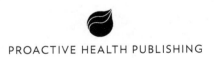

PROACTIVE HEALTH PUBLISHING

Proactive Health Publishing
1407 116th Ave NE Suite 104
Bellevue, WA 98004
www.proactivehealthnd.com

Ordering Information:
Please contact Proactive Health Publishing: Tel: 206-607-2708; Fax: 206-858-9710 or visit www.proactivehealthnd.com.

Printed in the United States of America

Publisher's Cataloging-in-Publication Data
Names: Zinkov, Elena, 1985-
Title: Crave reset : a breakthrough guide for mastering the psychology and physiology of cravings / Dr. Elena Zinkov, ND.
Description: Bellevue, WA : Proactive Health Publishing, 2018. | Includes bibliographical references and index. | Summary: Guides the reader in building new neurological pathways to help create healthy, medically sound and enduring behaviors using nutrition, mindfulness and exercise.
Identifiers: LCCN 2018939771 | ISBN 9781732096004 (hardcover) | ISBN 9781732096011 (pbk.) | ISBN 9781732096028 (Epub) | ISBN 9781732096035 (MOBI)
Subjects: LCSH: Compulsive eating -- Treatment. | Diet -- Psychological aspects. | Human physiology. | Metabolism   -- Regulation. | Nutrition. | BISAC: HEALTH & FITNESS / Diet & Nutrition / Weight Loss. | HEALTH & FITNESS /   Healthy Living. | SELF-HELP / Compulsive Behavior / General.
Classification: LCC RA784.Z56 2018 (print) | LCC RA784 (ebook) | DDC 613.2--dc23
LC record available at https://lccn.loc.gov/2018939771

First Edition

14 13 12 11 10 / 10 9 8 7 6 5 4 3 2 1

"Let food be thy medicine and medicine be thy food."
—HIPPOCRATES

To Stanislav and Slava,
you are my why.

MEDICAL DISCLAIMER

This book contains information intended to help the readers become better informed consumers of health care. It is presented as general advice on health care. Always consult your doctor for your individual needs. Before beginning any new exercise program, it is recommended that you seek medical advice from your personal physician. This book is not intended to be a substitute for the medical advice of a licensed physician, nor is it meant to diagnose or treat. The reader should consult with their doctor in any matters relating to his/her health.

Contents

Introduction

"The first wealth is health."
— RALPH WALDO EMERSON

Just because you can eat a whole cake doesn't mean you should. I had this realization after I had eaten yet another carrot cake. Even though I had started the day with laps in the pool and finished the training day with a sixty-mile bike ride, eating a six-inch carrot cake in one sitting got me thinking that I possibly had a problem with sugar.

I was raised as a competitive athlete, started playing competitive tennis when I was nine, and, as a teenager, spent countless hours on and off the court pursuing my dream of becoming a professional athlete. Because no one in my family really knew anything about nutrition, I found myself eating things that seemed right and, of course, pleasurable for a teenager – Corn Pops for breakfast, Milano cookies dipped in milk for lunch, Mountain Dew for water, a chocolate milk shake in the middle of practice, and a bag of peanuts during art class before an afternoon session of tennis.

For someone who played six to nine hours five days a week and stayed up until 1 a.m. doing homework for a very demanding private school, this was malnutrition. Even though my body did not show it—I was a lean, mean, fighting machine—I was falling asleep during class, had skin breakouts and digestive issues, and would find myself hungry during workouts.

In my early twenties, as I got burnt out in tennis and shifted my focus to other endurance sports like running, triathlons, and climbing, I still maintained some of my old habits of relying on sugar for fuel. I could easily throw down a carrot cake at the end of a training session or go through a loaf of bread with peanut butter and jelly.

Even though I had been able to get away with eating processed foods earlier in my life, my bad habits were catching up to me, and I knew something had to change. I began to ask the same questions that people ask me today: "Why do I crave what I crave?" and, most importantly, "What can I do about it?"

This began my love affair with finding sweet-tooth and salt-craving alternatives as well as focusing on the underlying factors that were predisposing me to overindulge.

As I was trying to change my diet, I was also facing the decision of what I wanted to do professionally with my life. I had just graduated from the University of Washington Foster School of Business, was working part-time at a commercial real estate company, and taught yoga in the evenings. My extensive background in sports made my day to day activities really mundane and, as I would say, "not very thrilling." I wanted to heal myself and then help others find their path to better health. Now that sounded more exciting.

Science had never been my strong point, so I was in for a treat when I enrolled into pre-med classes with the intention of getting into medical school. During one of my lectures, my physiology professor mentioned something about a vegan donut. One of my classmates said, "Well, it's gotta be healthy; it's vegan." The professor grinned and replied, "Sugar is sugar whether it's vegan or not." This was yet another moment of insight for a future to be doctor. My professor just happened to be on faculty at a school for naturopathic medicine, so when it came to deciding between conventional medical school or natural medicine, he helped me understand the difference between the two and discover what resonated with my intention to help people live truly healthy lives.

Most people these days are frustrated that their health care provider does not spend enough time with them to understand their real issues and does not provide the quality of care that they seek. Naturopathic medicine emphasizes treating the whole person rather than symptoms and emphasizes getting to the root cause of illness. Naturopathic physicians also follow a certain hierarchy of treatment to ensure that foundations of health are met first, such as diet and lifestyle, before higher intervention therapies are considered. My personal journey to overcome sugar addiction has greatly contributed to my desire to help people overcome their own addictions through understanding the root cause and source of addictions and has provided powerful tools and strategies to overcome them.

Cravings are a natural and inherent part of being human. This is our body's way of communicating with us, and it has an evolutionary and genetic component. But cravings also have a way of distracting us from the world around us. In this book, I will walk you through the basic science of food cravings. I will explain why we have cravings and, most importantly, how to manage them and live the ultimate life, crave free.

Everyone gets cravings for different reasons. This is why every chapter in this book has something new to offer, a different perspective and reason for cravings. While most books focus on one or two reasons, such as nutrient deficiencies (the famous correlation between magnesium and chocolate craving) or emotional eating (definitely a big reason!), I take the naturopathic and total body approach to cravings and address everything from genetics, hormones, brain health, and gut health to environmental influences.

In my own experience, I discovered that I was genetically predisposed to craving sugar and that I would have to work a little harder to stay away from it. I also found that I was tired from studying and training so much, that I ate foods that created all sorts of chaos in the gut, and that I was experiencing symptoms of a low-functioning thyroid. The reason I craved the cake and had the mindset to eat the whole thing was due to multiple factors, all of which needed to be addressed in order to gain a healthy mind and body.

It is essential to have a whole-body approach when dealing with food cravings. Whatever reason lies behind your cravings, this book has got you covered. Each chapter dives into either the science, physiology, or psychology of cravings. At the end of each chapter, exercises provide insight and tips on living a crave-free life. As you read along, you will be able to understand the messages behind your cravings and learn how to respond to them in the most gentle and effective way that won't leave you feeling irritated or frustrated. My intention is for you to be able to lift the fog and see more clearly past the nagging need to indulge.

To entice you even further: overcoming cravings for sugar and other foods can help you get a grasp on other destructive behaviors in your life. The link between all destructive behaviors is the pleasure-seeking nature of our brains, which manifests itself in our habits. Naturally, anything that brings us pleasure is addicting, so I will spend the first couple of chapters talking about the science behind cravings, and I will shed light on two very important neural pathways that motivate this negative behavior.

Cravings can be challenging to overcome. At times you may have felt desperate and out of control. One of the most important things we will dive into is the evolution of humans around food. The information presented here comes at a time in our history when we are literally living to eat rather than eating to live. Food in general is still scarce in most parts of the world and in some parts of our country, but generally speaking, we live in a time of abundance when we can walk into any grocery or convenience store and have at it. There's everything we need to satisfy our internal cookie monster! Understanding the evolutionary component behind the strong urge to indulge and overindulge will be one of the first steps we'll take on the journey to a crave-free life. Even now, take a moment and reflect on how easy or challenging it was for your ancestors to have access to what you have today.

From an evolutionary perspective, certain parts of our brains have not evolved that much and drive our instinctive behavior purely out of survival. If we go back to Paleolithic times when saber-toothed tigers were a threat and foods containing sugar and fat were scarce (and did not exist in present day form), we'd see that being able to run away and have a meal were life's essentials. Nowadays, we run away from our bosses, cell phones, spouses, to-do lists, and anything else that drives our stress response, because as far as the brain is concerned, all of those are in the same category as the saber-toothed tiger. To make the situation worse, we also fuel our stress response with the foods that used to be scarce but are now at our fingertips. I will guide you through several chapters that look into social behavior around food and will provide you with tools to help you succeed regardless of the environment you find yourself in.

Something I encourage you to do before you jump into resetting your food cravings is to consider what other negative habits go along with the foods that you desire the most. This can be insightful to think about, as foods rich in fat, sugar, and salt target the same reward pathways in our brain that are also targeted by alcohol, nicotine, and behaviors like shopping and gambling. Let's get one thing straight, however, before we go any further—I am not talking about having a glass of wine occasionally, doing some retail therapy once in a while, or taking a trip to Vegas and throwing some money at the gambling machines. I wouldn't consider those negative behaviors or habits, unless they were destroying or negatively impacting your health and life.

So for a moment, consider: Which habits come in pairs for you? You may reach for a cigarette when you get stressed out, but the brain knows that aside from nicotine, a bag of salty potato chips will do just the trick. At some point, we are either trading one habit for another that is just as equally hurtful (but feels so good at the moment!), or we are partaking in all of them throughout the day: a cookie in the break room, a smoke break, and a cocktail after a long day at work. What all of these habits have in common is that they activate the pleasure pathways in the brain and alter the neurochemistry to make you feel addicted to the behaviors that provide comfort, security, and a brief moment of pleasure. Don't we all wish eating kale would have this effect?

Something else to think about is how these habits manifest in your life and what they hold you back from accomplishing. At a time when many people work from home, and everyone wishes they had an extra two hours during the day to get things done, distractions zap those special minutes that, in turn, equal the two or more hours we want. I am guilty of this, and, believe it or not, writing this book was so eye opening for me, considering just how disciplined and focused I had to be to get this done and share the message with you. I can't tell you how many times the whole-carrot-cake-eating-Elena wanted to come out and visit. But I couldn't allow that. Allowing that would have taken me away from a purpose that meant so much to me, and I couldn't let a craving or an impulse dictate the course of my day, especially as I only had a few minutes to write at a time. Such is the fate of a new mom juggling a medical practice and a business.

As our attention spans get shorter and work days get longer, we are on a constant hunt for activities that will bring us pleasure, something that will numb the pain of a long meeting or work day or maybe serve as a distraction from the present moment. I have an absolute fascination with the human brain. It can solve puzzles and complex problems, innovate, and provide Nobel Prize solutions. Yet when given the choice, it prefers to take the road most travelled and will do whatever necessary to take the easiest route to get you to a place of comfort, because at the root of making any decision is pleasure, fulfillment, and certainty, as opposed to pain, dissatisfaction, and uncertainty. When faced with a tough task that requires all of our attention, we rarely respond, "Yes! This is what I've been waiting for!" For most of us, it's usually more like, "Dang it! Why me?" Although we are capable of solving complex problems, we would rather deal with issues on a simpler level, where there is little pain, because biologically, we are hardwired to steer away from pain and toward pleasure.

Mindfulness, or lack of it, is at the root of the important decisions we make during the day. Some guided meditations start by asking you to imagine your brain as an untamed stallion, frolicking in the fields, bouncing all over the place, and galloping whichever way the wind blows. This description of our minds is not far from the truth, as we are constantly doing mental gymnastics. Our computer screens or iPhones have a gazillion screens open at any point time, we are watching YouTube videos while trying to focus on a task at hand, including eating, and some of us are talking on the phone while at the same time holding a baby. That's a lot of information to process for the brain, which is designed to focus on one thing at a time. When asked to pull it together and focus, the brain almost doesn't know how. Having a been a personal victim of multitasking, I will show you how you can become more mindful in your day-to-day activities to reap the greatest rewards in health, relationships, and personal and professional growth.

The beauty of the whole process of getting to know what you're craving, why you're craving, and what it's truly keeping you away from achieving, is that we get to know ourselves at a deeper level. Many of us use food as a coping mechanism and something that will bring instant gratification. Some us may not even be sure why we reach for certain foods in the first place, which is a frustrating place to be. In any case, cravings are our partners in crime, instigating impulsive behavior and overriding any conscious effort to stop. They give us the gratifying experience of pleasure followed by remorse over what happened. You can take charge of the habits that have previously consumed you and deprived you of the joy of being in the present moment. Just as I have helped hundreds of people overcome their negative habits around their personal cravings, I'll show in this book how you can have the same success as well.

Our cravings are a result of an intricate web of genetics, neurology, psychology, endocrinology, environment, and gut-brain relationship, all of which are responsible for the pesky cravings for sugar, fat, caffeine, and salt, which fill our pantries, cabinets, meeting spaces, and, most importantly, our misled minds. But in its inherent and intelligent wisdom, the body communicates to us through an array of symptoms, and cravings are one of the ways we receive the message. As you go through this book, your mind will be blown by how much information is contained in your cravings!

Connecting with your body's natural wisdom and accepting its message in the form of a craving can be eye opening and healing and will lead you to a path of better health. Ignoring the message can leave you feeling distracted, frustrated, and "hangry" and break you down instead of building you up. Addictions, including cravings for food, are a major distraction and barrier to the flow of our day-to-day attention, focus, and productivity.

To help you get the big picture before you get started, consider the basic questions below to evaluate the nature, source, and quality of your cravings:

- How would you describe your cravings? When do they usually happen? What triggers them?

- When did you first start having cravings? Have you always had them, or can you pinpoint a time in your life when they started to appear more often?

- Aside from cravings, how is your energy throughout the day? How is your mood, digestion, and anything else pertaining to your everyday experience? For women, it is important to understand and note how this may change depending on where they are in the cycle.

- What are your cravings preventing you from doing, achieving, and feeling?

In each chapter, I help you understand the source of cravings and provide valuable exercises to start rewiring your brain and your whole body in the process, to reveal a brand spanking new you.

You will find tasty recipes throughout the chapters, and there are plenty more at the end of the book. Included is also my popular 14-day Crave Reset™ Sugar Cleanse, which I call a "palette cleanser." It's not limiting, and you'll see how you can still find sweetness naturally. The recipes and the cleanse have been lifesavers for me and everyone I have helped over the years and continue to be my personal go-to's during frazzled times, at holidays, or when my body needs a tune up.

It's time to end your personal battle with cravings and start reclaiming your personal health, happiness, and peace of mind. I sincerely wish you all the courage, determination, patience, and compassion for yourself as you begin the journey to better health.

In Health,

Dr. Elena Zinkov
Bellevue, WA
2018

CHAPTER 1
The Science Behind Cravings

*"No one can exert cognitive inhibition, willpower, over a biochemical
drive that goes on every minute, of every day, of every year."*

– Dr. Robert H. Lustig

Anyone can be addicted to sugar. In my case, I was an athlete who
did not have to worry, from a weight perspective, about the type
of calories going into my body. For me, it was just important to
get in as much fuel as I could and when I could. It was my natural
curiosity about why I was so inclined to eat certain foods more
than others when given the choice that led me to explore the
science behind cravings. Although we hear about the addicting
nature of food, we don't realize just how addicting it can be until
we try to give it up.

I once had a conversation with one of my patients, who
stated that she needed sugar. When I asked what made her
think she needed sugar, she told me that when she tried
removing it from her diet, she felt awful! Her assumption
was that if she felt like crap without it, it was necessary for
her to continue, including via cookies and in coffee or tea. I
explained that what she had been experiencing for the two
weeks after removing sugar were withdrawal symptoms or
a "sugar hangover," which is worse than the other common
hangover.

The American Heart Association has put out warnings against
the amount of sugar added to the typical American diet, and the

rest of the world is catching on. If we look historically to the 1700s, we find that sugar consumption was around two kilograms per person in average per year. By 1870, that number drastically increased to twenty-five kilograms a year, and nowadays, the average American consumes about sixty kilograms of sugar a year. That's a staggering 132 pounds of pure sugar that makes its way into our diet each year in a form of soda, candy bars, cereal, cakes, cookies, and anything else it's sprinkled on. If we think about a pound of sugar equaling 1,775 calories, that equates to 234,300 calories!

Not only is that a whole lot of empty calories, but sugar is also considered to be super toxic. My patient who was trying to give up the sugar was not only experiencing the addicting nature of sugar, but she was also having symptoms of detoxing from sugar, including headaches, fatigue, and irritability. If she had continued with her sugar detox program and had gotten the right support and resources, she would have kicked the habit and would have continued to enjoy the numerous health benefits. At the end of this chapter, I'll guide you through a basic "junk food audit" to see if you are someone who experiences some of the symptoms of sugar or processed food overload.

Let's get to the important questions of why sugar and junk food cravings are so hard to beat and why so many people resort to old eating habits.

Cravings can bring about a whole lot of trouble for even the most conscious of healthy eaters. It's extremely challenging to stand against the nagging need to eat something that makes you salivate just at the idea of thinking about the food you want. Willpower may get you through a trip to the grocery store or Thanksgiving dinner, but you'll need a better strategy to help you manage cravings long term.

Next time you find yourself with an empty pint of ice cream consider the following: a growing amount of evidence shows that foods high in sugar and fat, like candy, cookies, and cheesecake (all the items typically found in work break-rooms and home pantries), are addicting, comparable to drug addiction and alcoholism. Just how addicting is sugar? Brain studies have shown that cocaine and sugar target the same pleasure pathways in the brain, but sugar is eight times more addicting! Not double or triple but eight times more addicting!

Once you understand that sugar is just as addictive, if not more, than tobacco, alcohol, and others substances, you'll see why getting off sugar can be so agonizing. At the root of the problem is our mind and its intricate neural pathways, which become so strong that we can't walk through the baked goods section without picking up anything or drive home from the store with the box of cookies still intact.

According to *Obesity Research and Clinical Practice Journal*, food cravings are comparable to drug addiction, based on the similar production of neurotransmitters, mainly serotonin. Carbohydrate consumption – and sugar is a form of a carbohydrate – affects the serotonin-releasing neurons in our brain, which normally control the amount of serotonin neurotransmitter that gets released into the bloodstream, based on carbohydrate intake. The release of serotonin is what instantly gives you a gratified feeling.[1] Further fueling the craving mind, serotonin is involved in basic body functions like sleep onset, pain sensitivity, blood pressure regulation, and mood. This helps to explain why, when we are in physical or emotional pain, feel depressed or agitated, or can't fall asleep, we reach for carbohydrates to give us a quick fix and temporary "relief." Think of a time in your life when you were getting very little sleep. What were you craving throughout the day?

The similarity between sugar and carbohydrate addiction to substances like nicotine is proven by research and helps us understand why sugar consumption is a hard habit to kick. Nicotine, like carbohydrates, increases brain serotonin secretion, while nicotine withdrawal has the opposite effect. Why do most people gain weight when they quit smoking? Because most resort to overconsumption of feel-good carbohydrates and fats to make up for the loss of feel-good serotonin.

Let's take a look at a common snack loved by many: chocolate. Cacao in chocolate is not the source of the problem, rather it is the combination of cacao and the sugar that usually accompanies it. Cacao contains what is known as an anandamide, or "chocolate amphetamine," that creates feelings of excitement and alertness. A common recreational drug, cannabis, also contains anandamide. Chocolate in its processed form not only has a similar effect as cannabis but also creates the feel-good sensation from sugar similar to other drugs noted. This is not meant to take away from the pleasure of having a piece of chocolate but rather to provide insight into why some have a hard time putting the chocolate bar down. Don't shoot the messenger here! I love a good chocolate bar once in a while, but I will also provide recipes throughout this book to help you use raw cacao in a naturally sweet form so that you can tame the sweet tooth and give yourself a boost at the same time.

Sugar, fat, and salt are not the only bad guys on our list when it comes to processed foods. Most refined products usually contain some sort of preservatives or additives in order to extend shelf life, add a nice color, and, of course, make your taste buds go wild. The addictive nature of processed foods is highlighted by Dr. Russell Blaylock, a neurosurgeon, who describes the similarity between drugs and the addictive nature of food additives, "Many processed foods contain monosodium glutamate (MSG) and other sources of glutamate — a powerful, taste-enhancing amino acid. When foods taste this good, they activate the pleasure centers in the brain, which are also regulated by glutamate neurotransmission. This can produce the same powerful addiction impulse as cocaine and other addictive drugs. So, we have a dual force, a sense of hunger and a sense of addiction, driving our appetites."

That last sentence reminds me of one my friends who, a long time ago, commented on the addictive nature of French fries from a popular, global fast-food company: "I don't know what they sprinkle on those fries besides salt. It's as if they toss them in some cocaine right before they hand them to you. I know they are terrible for me, but I can't resist the taste."

Fries, burgers, or any other fried food for that matter contains some levels of taste enhancing glutamate, and your hooked brain lets you know when it starts to miss it. I am shocked, stunned, bewildered, stupefied, and surprised by the amount of traffic formed from cars rolling into the most popular fast food chain restaurants. I won't mention any names, because I don't stand a chance against their behemoth lawyers. But I will say that, at this point in time, when we have access to so much information on health and wellness, and when we know what those foods are to doing to us from the inside out, I see an extraordinarily large number of people opting for drive-throughs rather than the salad bar.

Back to my patient who mentioned she "needed" sugar. In her mind, it truly did feel like a need or a must have—something she could not live without. She realized how much her energy depended on sugar and processed carbohydrates. I changed the types and quality of carbohydrates she was eating to help her feel full and satisfied. I provided her with many different recipes that she could make in no time and take with her to work or school. I encouraged her to move her body multiple times a day, and she even committed to weekly personal training sessions at a gym near her work. My patient was glowing by the end of our journey together. To top it off, she was about to embark on her next career move, and she was happy to do so in a healthier body and with a crave free mind.

The total body approach that I used with my patient is something I teach in this book so that you can stop switching from one drug or habit to another. It's time to build new neurological pathways to help create healthy and long-lasting behaviors using nutrition, mindfulness, physical exercise, and the application of new habits.

Some of you are already at your pantry throwing away anything that has processed sugar or fat in it, because you've just had enough. I encourage you to read on and understand why sugar and fats are so appealing to us from a historical and ancestral perspective, what are some possible health conditions related to over-indulgence, and who or what are the culprits in your present environment that are preventing you from kicking the habit.

➤ CHAPTER 1 EXERCISE: The Junk Food Audit

Before we get into more of the juicy details and learn to understand our cravings, I want you to get a baseline for where you are now and where you want to be. Below is a list of questions that will evaluate just how much food cravings are involved in your life. The first step is to recognize the problem. Every chapter that follows will address all the layers of cravings so that you can find the most appropriate path for yourself.

The following questionnaire is a shorter, simplified version of the Yale Food Addiction Scale. When answering this questionnaire, think about your eating habits for the past year and how certain foods like ice cream, candy, cake, salty snacks like chips, and fatty foods like steak and French fries have a daily impact on your emotional and physical well-being. Be kind to yourself as you go through the list of questions, knowing that you are taking a great step toward understanding where the issue lies. Most people do not voice their concerns about addictive behavior. You're not alone!

Please note that this is not meant to diagnose or treat but simply to create a baseline marker and provide insight. The actual Yale Food Addiction Scale is much more comprehensive and is used as a clinical tool for physicians.

On a scale of 0-5, 0 being not at all and 5 being often, rate the following:

1. Do you wake up feeling tired most mornings?
2. Do you get headaches or feel agitated if you avoid coffee?
3. Do you experience headaches or irritability when limiting processed foods?
4. Do you have more than one packaged food item per day (chips, bars, etc)
5. Have you found yourself in a difficult situation and your

---

immediate response was to grab something sweet, salty, or crunchy?

6.   Do you tend to isolate yourself when you feel anxious, sad, or depressed?

7.   Do you experience late night snacking?

8.   Do you have a hard time saying no to co-worker's treats?

9.   More often than not, do you find yourself finishing a bag of your favorite snack without even noticing?

10. Do you snack at your work desk, in your car, or anytime really?

11. Do you frequently eat even when you're not hungry?

12. Do you think about food constantly?

13. Are you using food to escape from feelings or the present moment?

14. Have you found yourself not being able to stop eating a certain food?

15. Do you avoid certain social or professional engagements due to concern of overeating?

16. Even when you eat a "pleasurable" food, do you find that these foods don't make you feel better?

17. Do you consume certain foods, sweet and salty in particular, to prevent certain feelings or emotions?

18. Does food in general cause distress?

19. Do you have the urge to eat certain foods when you cut back on them?

Add up the total for your ratings. If you scored 14 or more on the questions, then you can benefit from the next chapters, which look into the fundamental causes for food cravings that includes neurotransmitter deficiencies, hormone imbalances, digestive health, and even social circumstances—everything and anything that can make you rate high on the questionnaire. Come back to these questions as you go through the book to see how the answers change as you apply some of the lessons, strategies, and recipes.

CHAPTER 2
A Case for Evolution and Role of Genetics

"I'm a food addict. We all are. Our brains are biologically driven to seek and devour high-calorie, fatty foods. The difference is that I have learned how to control those primitive parts of my brain. Anyone can do this if they know how."

—Dr. Mark Hyman

Some of us are genetically much more prone to sugar and other food addictions than others. I have observed this in my private practice over the years as I have seen some people more capable of kicking the habit compared with others. One of the dominating factors in food addiction is that every individual has a preprogrammed pleasure threshold that is dictated by the previously mentioned reward center in our brain. Some individuals require little stimulus to be content, while others reach for addicting habits uncontrollably, or more than others, to get the same effect.

One of my patients came to me because she was struggling with both the quality of food she was eating as well as the quantity. "I will have the best intentions," she said, "then it's like a switch will go off and I find myself finishing my plate and reaching for my husband's." Some words she used to describe her cravings and her need to overindulge were: overpowering, strong, beyond her, impulsive, and overwhelming. I am sure anyone who's had their struggle with cravings can relate.

I have often found my patients struggling to make sense of

their food cravings – the powerful urge to consume sugary snacks in the break room or high fat snacks from the vending machine or to splurge on the happy hour menu after work. Our sweet tooth, along with a gamut of other gnarly cravings like salt and processed fat, is a result not only of our physiology and lifestyle but also of our genetics and ancestry. The medical community is in joint agreement that we are naturally hardwired to reach for readily available processed foods due to the scarcity of calories that our ancestors previously experienced. How many of us catch our breakfast or wander around the forest picking berries these days? A very small percentage worldwide.

From an evolutionary point of view "our brains haven't evolved as fast as our food environment. The human brain evolved over 2.5 million years ago. And with the exception of the last ten-thousand years, people only ate animals they could hunt and wild-plants they could gather," says Dr. Hyman in his article "How to Rewire Your Brain to End Food Cravings."[9]

The combination of easy access to drive-through restaurants and deli counters together with less daily movement in comparison to previous generations has drastically affected our perception of food and has altered our physiology on multiple levels. It's no wonder that our minds and bodies are confused given the amount of choices in any given store. A label that says "organic" these days doesn't mean a whole lot, as there are so many other factors to consider, including the manufacturing and processing of food. Of course, get organic when you can, but you get the point: Look further at the label and maybe even research your favorite brands.

I am not exaggerating when I say that cravings are an intricate web of multiple factors. But genetics can influence how frequently we eat, the quantity of food we take in at any given time, and our food preferences. Besides our natural predisposition to eat highly caloric foods from an evolutionary perspective, our genetic composition can influence everything from how sensitive our taste buds are to sweets to how easily we curb our appetites. Have you ever noticed how some people can't live without a slice of cake, whereas others could care less about it? I'll show you how you can become the person who can easily say no thanks to the cake. It's part genetics and part rewiring our taste buds and our brains to change what we crave—you can only blame your parents for so much!

A study presented at the European Society of Human Genetics found that people's preferences for foods like bacon, coffee, blue cheese, dark chocolate, and (everyone's favorite) broccoli can be linked to certain genes. Based on the research presented, this also applies to the amount of sugar someone is inclined to eat. Out of the thousands of genes we have, a few are responsible for our food preferences and aversions as well as our ability to regulate hunger, mood, and appetite. It's time to get to know these genes and take control over how they present themselves in our day to day life.

Let's start with the basics of taste and how taste is influenced from the genetic perspective. There are five tastes recognized by humans: sweet, bitter, sour, salty, and umami or earthy taste (think about foods containing miso, mushrooms, and cheese). Research has shown that food preference and intake is highly influenced by the sweet and bitter taste of food. When you're looking at a menu or a buffet, which foods seem more or less appealing? Individuals who have an enhanced perception of bitter taste will tend to avoid certain fruit and vegetables, while preferring sweet and high fat foods instead—all of which can be determined by your genes.[48]

The gene responsible for affecting an individual's perception of bitter taste in food is called TAS2R38. It affects an individual's ability to enjoy healthy foods that contain bitter compounds, such as broccoli and kale, while finding sweets particularly satisfying. A variation of the TAS2R38 gene can also increase the number of taste buds responsible for detecting bitter compounds. Individuals with this variation and its added sensitivity to bitter compounds are often referred to as super-tasters. [49] The solution is to search for fruits and vegetables that are both healthy and pleasing to the palate. In doing some personal research and building a rich recipe database, you will be able to put together a diet plan that is healthy and, most importantly, sustainable for you.

In the study of genetics and the tendency to overindulge in sweets, one gene that has been heavily researched is the gene that codes for a glucose transporter protein found in cell membranes. It's called GLUT2. The name is deceiving, as it has nothing to do with the gluteal muscles or your "glutes." GLUT2 is one of the most important proteins and helps facilitate the movement of glucose from our blood into our cells, thus helping keep blood sugar stable. Some individuals can move glucose more efficiently, which is one of many reasons why not everyone has the same tendency to crave sugar or sweet foods. But since you are reading this book, chances are you are likely experiencing heightened sugar cravings and are looking for solutions. Knowing that we may have a tendency to overindulge given our genetics is step one. Doing our part to control sugar intake as part of our long-term health strategy is step two. As we go through the other genes and discover how they impact our behavior around food, pay attention to which genes you have the hardest time with—at the end of the chapter, I'll provide a detailed plan for how to minimize their impact to help you break through the craving cycle.

As I showed earlier with my patient who was hungry for her husband's plate, our genetics impact not only the types of foods we crave but also the quantity of food we consume. While some individuals have a hard time making healthy food choices, others struggle with eating too much, and some have difficulty with both. These individual differences in eating behavior are partly due to genetics. One example is the FTO gene, which has a direct effect on the activity of the hunger-signaling hormone known as ghrelin. Think of the noise that your stomach makes when you're hungry, and you won't forget!

Your genotype for the FTO gene can be associated with low, normal, or high levels of the hunger stimulating hormone. Normal levels suggest that a person has a normal level of difficulty in controlling appetite and hunger. High levels of ghrelin, however, suggest that a person has a hard time controlling hunger, quantity, and quality of food consumed. This provides insight into why some people have an easier time preventing or avoiding the 'hangry' state, while others get trapped in an emotional rollercoaster that takes everyone in the vicinity for a ride.

My patient who had a hard time controlling her caloric intake was genetically predisposed to have higher than normal levels of ghrelin, and she did have difficulty controlling her appetite. However, there is plenty of research that shows the impact of diet, exercise, and lifestyle modifications on gene expression. Just as I helped my patient get her appetite under control regardless of her genetic make-up, I'll provide you with tips at the end of the chapter to help you do the same. But for now, let's take a look at other genes, particularly those that impact our mood around food.

Many of us eat for pleasure even when we are not hungry. In chapter one, I talked about the reason food is so addicting. It's because of the direct link to a key pleasure neurotransmitter, serotonin. But another neurotransmitter involved in mood and motivation, and one that's important in solidifying behavior around food, is dopamine. Dopamine receptors, coded by the DRD2 or D2 gene, play an important role in bringing pleasure and creating repetitive behavior around it. D2 must be turned on for us to experience the feelings of pleasure. The amino acid dopamine triggers activation of these receptors and creates the desired response. Sugar, along with other foods and drugs, increases dopamine production for the extent of the activity. Those who experience food addiction, partake in compulsive eating, and experience the tendency to gain weight may have fewer D2 dopamine receptors and need extra stimulation to experience pleasure.[50] MRI studies of both lean and obese teenagers found that teenagers whose brains didn't light up as much with stimulation in the dopamine reward centers were more likely to be obese and gain weight later and were more likely to have the D2 gene that coded for fewer dopamine receptors [51].

The D2 gene variation of the dopamine receptor has been correlated with reduced dopamine receptor density in the brain.

Individuals with fewer of these receptors may be more susceptible to substance abuse along with overconsumption of food.

In addition, some studies have shown how drugs can modulate this defective dopamine reward response. In one study, naltrexone, an opioid blocker, which blocks the effects of heroin and morphine in the brain, was used with sugar addicts. When this drug was taken, it prevented addicts from experiencing the pleasure they normally got from consuming sugar, and they ended up craving and eating less. A similar effect has been noted with substances like nicotine and drugs like Ritalin used in ADHD management.

There is no doubt that in order for us to make better food decisions, we need to be in a better mood. The reason I believe it is so important to understand the role of genetics is because when we cultivate awareness regarding the issue, we then have the power to do something about it. Over the last few years, one of the most important genes that has taken center stage in the medical community is the MTHFR gene. This is due, in part, to the fabulous work of a fellow naturopathic physician, Dr. Ben Lynch, who has dedicated his career to helping people thrive and make the best of their genetics.

MTHFR is a gene that provides instructions for making an enzyme called methylenetetrahydrofolate reductase (MTHFR), which takes folic acid from food and converts it into an active methyl-folate form that your body can use. Methyl-folate travels through the blood stream and delivers the methyl group to a variety of important biochemical pathways. MTHFR gene mutation results in a problem that involves poor methylation and enzyme production, so that the body cannot convert folic acid into the proper active form. There are two main mutations that can occur and affect genes referred to as MTHFR A1298C and MTHFR C677T. Mutations can occur on different locations of these genes, and every person is affected differently. Some have hardly any symptoms, while others inherit a host of health issues.

Why is methylation such an important process, and how is it detrimental to our health and well-being?

Methylation is involved in cell regeneration and repair, gene expression, B vitamin metabolism, and regulation of the key neurotransmitters serotonin and dopamine, which in turn affect mood and behavior. Methylation is also a very important step in optimizing our immune function, controlling inflammation, aiding fat metabolism in the liver, and promoting detoxification. Mutation in the MTHFR gene can have a significant negative impact on our health, as it can cause up to a 70% reduction in the MTHFR enzyme production, which means less folate gets converted to methyl-folate, putting a wrench into the whole methylation process. From what we know about MTFHR, its mutation can contribute to higher risk of cardiovascular disease, weight gain, and abnormal immune function, and can increase symptoms of depression, as it impacts neurotransmitter function.

As you can see, MTHFR is involved in so many processes that I cannot not talk about mood and behavior as they relate to food without talking about MTHFR. There are many things you can do to help identify and manage MTHFR mutation. The first step is to identify if you, in fact, have a mutation of the gene. The 23andme genetic test is a good starting point and is a popular test that reveals more about your health than you would ever want to know. If you are looking to get a better sense of your food cravings, to learn about your predisposition in regard to appetite control and emotional eating, and to also see if you have low or normal MTHFR activity, then I recommend asking your healthcare provider if there is a genetic test that they use or recommend. In my private practice, I personally used Genovive's comprehensive nutrition, fitness, and behavior profile to help my patients get a clearer picture of their genetic make-up as it relates to nutrition, behavior, and fitness. You can find more information on my website by visiting proactivehealthnd.com/genetictesting. If you have already done a genetic test, and you know you have the mutation or decreased activity of the MTHFR enzyme, not to worry. At the end of the chapter, I will provide numerous solutions to help you improve and correct MTHFR activity for the most optimal health results!

We've covered a lot of ground in the world of genetics and food cravings. But before you start blaming your parents for the genes you inherited, I encourage you to consider the role your environment and lifestyle choices play in gene expression. After all, our environment and lifestyle can drastically impact which genes are expressed more than others, and most common illnesses are a result of both genetic predisposition and the surrounding environment.

Our environment can include the direct outer environment that we find ourselves in, such as family, work, and social. But it can also include the quality of the air we breathe and the toxins we are exposed to on a daily basis. Although I will talk more on the subject of work, family, and social circles in shaping our cravings, if you would like to learn more about genetics and how you can improve overall health, I encourage you to look into Dr. Lynch's book, *Dirty Genes*.

Even though genetics play an important role in shaping our minds, bodies, and behaviors, there is so much you can do to change how you respond to different stimuli in your environment and, as a result, change your health outcomes. At the end of this chapter, I provide you with strategies to help you manage emotional eating, conquer overeating, and learn better ways to manage your surrounding environment, even if you're not so genetically inclined.

►**CHAPTER 2 EXERCISE:** Top 5 Tips for Decreasing Hunger, Controlling Appetite, and Managing Emotional Eating:

#1 Appetite and Food Selection—Managing Hunger with the Right Foods

I mentioned the role of the FTO gene and how it can impact appetite control and hunger. Because this gene influences the activity of the hunger hormone ghrelin, too much activity can make it easy to overindulge when you don't really need to. There are simple ways that you can optimize your caloric intake, feel more satisfied in between meals, and fend off hunger.

Protein and fiber rich foods provide feelings of fullness and take much longer to digest than foods high in processed carbohydrates. Plan for each meal to have some source of protein, and you'll notice just how much more satisfied and less deprived you feel. Loading up on protein is important for the synthesis of our feel-good neurotransmitters, so including protein with every meal, vegetarian or animal, can mean better moods and better decisions around food. For fiber, load up on fibrous foods, such as non-starchy vegetables and greens. Not only will this leave you feeling full, but it will also provide a bonus for your digestion.

#2 Eating for Pleasure—Keep Emotions at Bay

One of the reasons cravings can be hard to beat is because of the pleasure that we associate with food. Genetically, we want to engage in behaviors that bring pleasure, but in modern times this can be a real problem. I talked about the DRD2 gene and the role that dopamine plays in influencing our moods and decisions around food.

If you've ever wondered why one slice of cake or one serving of ice cream is never enough, the answer is that a variation in this gene can result in a reduced sensation of satisfaction or pleasure and can also contribute to increased impulsivity and a preference for foods with higher calories.

One of the best things you can do is find foods that not only taste good but are also good for you. Use the recipes found throughout this book to help you get started, because they contain healthy sources of protein, fat, and carbohydrates and contain sweetness from natural sources like honey and maple syrup. Part of retraining your palette and shifting away from the processed foods that you're used to is introducing foods that are nutrient dense and have multiple health benefits.

You may find that initially, you still slip and resort to old habits. But trust that over time your old habits will be replaced with a new and healthier way of eating that is fulfilling, pleasurable, and guilt free.

Another major point to address is blood sugar and maintaining optimal levels throughout the day. This is crucial, because most impulsive decisions are made when blood sugar levels are low, which creates a sense of irritability, frustration, and fatigue and contributes to making irrational decisions. Keeping blood sugar stable can easily be done in multiple ways:

1. By making sure your meals contain good sources of protein, fiber, and complex carbohydrates, such as whole grains and vegetables.
2. By not skipping meals and not allowing blood sugar to drop so that you don't enter the "no turnaround zone."
3. Eating within sixty to ninety minutes of waking to balance blood sugar, which tends to spike first thing in the morning as a result of our stress hormone cortisol trying to get us amped up for the day.
4. There are also ways you can increase levels of dopamine naturally. This is covered in detail in the next chapter, where I discuss food and supplement support for best results.

#3 Change Your Surrounding Environment— Remove Obstacles to Your Cravings

Genetics play a big part in who we are, but our environment shapes us literally and figuratively more than we can comprehend. Throw out, donate, or give to your frenemies anything that is fueling your cravings. The more we give in to our cravings, the harder it becomes to give them up.

Whenever I take my patients through an extensive elimination challenge or a cleanse, or when we are simply cleaning things up, I ask them to restock their refrigerator and pantry with whole foods—minimally processed items, such as lean meats, eggs, fruits, vegetables, berries, nuts, and whole grains.

If you're planning on dining out, choose a place where you know you can find healthy menu items. If you're going to a baseball game or a happy hour with friends and healthy options will not be as readily available, have a snack or meal beforehand to last until your next meal. I can't tell you how often I hear complaints of work happy hours and weekend football parties that throw people off and how easily preventable that is! You can change your environment by being in the captain's seat of decision- making. We may not be able to control which genes we inherit, but we can control where and what we eat, who is in our social circle, and how we choose to respond to different stressors and stimuli, all of which can impact gene expression.

One of my patients, an avid outdoors woman, loved long hikes followed by fancy outings involving wine, champagne, and weekend restaurant runs. She had been recently divorced and was enjoying spending time outside and living the life with her girlfriends. She came to my office desperately trying to lose weight, claiming she had tried everything else. After our extensive conversation regarding her habits, she realized that even though she was eating healthy on weekdays and was exercising daily, her weekend rituals were sabotaging everything she did during the week.

We talked about dining out after her long, weekend hikes, as she still wanted to enjoy the company of her girlfriends without jeopardizing her health and waistline. We discussed how she could make better decisions during the week when going out with colleagues from work, and she learned just how much her social environment and the behavior of her closest friends was affecting her choices.

Just as you did a junk food audit in chapter one, do a personal environment audit. See what is currently happening in your family, social, and work environments that could use improvement.

#4 Fix Your Energy Gap—Address the Root Cause

As a physician, I see people battling fatigue all the time in many different contexts. When you're tired and your energy is off balance, sugar and other processed foods are much more pleasing to the eye and the palate. The gap in energy can be due to various reasons, many of which I will address later, but since we're on the subject of genetics, I'd like to shift attention to the MTHFR gene and its health implications. As I mentioned earlier, this gene plays an important role in how dietary folate is processed. Folate is a very important B vitamin involved in many metabolic processes, including energy production and mood regulation. A genetic mutation, which is more common these days and is often misdiagnosed, can mean that dietary folate, found in dark leafy greens, is not getting converted into its methylated bioavailable form. So even if you're eating the right foods, you may wonder why you're experiencing symptoms of poor energy, fatigue, irritability, and even weight gain.

If you do have symptoms of a MTHFR gene mutation, here are my top three tips that you can implement to help your body function more optimally:

1. Heal your gut: Optimize food breakdown and nutrient absorption. You want to get the most out of your nutrition. Improving digestion, removing food allergens, increasing elimination of toxins and waste, and balancing gut bacteria are all essential steps to creating a healthy digestive system. I will cover these important steps in the chapter that focuses on gut health.

2. Use the right supplements: With MTHFR mutation, having too much folate can be a problem, as it is not properly utilized by the body and builds up in the system. Symptoms of a build-up can include mood swings, irritability, gut upset, and sleeplessness. If you want to supplement with folic acid, or B12 for that matter, it's best to do so in the readily absorbable form or methylated form, since the body cannot methylate properly with an MTHFR mutation. This includes supplements like methyl folate and methyl B12. Consult your physician first before starting any new therapy and to have proper guidance on this journey!

3. Practice daily detox: Toxins found in water, air, and food can hinder the methylation process even in the healthiest of individuals, who don't have a mutation. To limit exposure, include grass fed meats, organic fruits and vegetables, and gluten-free grains to help with bowel movements and elimination. One of the best things you can do to increase elimination of daily accumulated toxins is to sweat. That's right: sweat, baby, sweat! Use the local hot yoga studio, go for a run, sweat in the gym, or hop into a sauna to open up the skin pores and help release toxins through sweat.

5 Consider Genetic Testing—Know What to Be Mindful Of

A genetic test can help you understand which genes are the biggest culprits for you and can also provide a customized nutrition, exercise, and lifestyle plan. The Genovive genetic test that I use in my private practice provides a complete breakdown of macronutrients—carbs, fat, and proteins—in optimal amounts specifically catered to every individual. The test also suggests ideal exercise intensity based on genetic predisposition, as well as information regarding behavior patterns around food and how to better manage them.

You don't have to complete this test in particular, as there are many tests out there. But do consult with your healthcare provider to find what works best for you or which test they would suggest. If you are interested in the testing that I do, visit proactivehealthnd.com/genetictesting to learn more. This is just one of many ways to get a clearer picture of what's behind your cravings and to help create a roadmap that is unique to you!

CHAPTER 3
Brain Chemistry and Addiction—
The Connection

"Excessive food intake may be explained more by dysfunction in the
reward circuitry than strictly dysfunction in the mechanisms
controlling feeding habits."

—CURRENT TOPICS IN BEHAVIORAL NEUROSCIENCE

In Latin, the word "addiction" is derived from a term
meaning "enslaved by." Anyone who has struggled to overcome
an addiction, whether to drugs or food, understands that this is a
very accurate description. Addiction involves craving something
so intensely that there is loss of control over its use despite adverse
consequences. The loss of control is, in part, due to changes in
brain chemistry—first by changing the way the brain registers
pleasure and then by changing other normal drives, such as
learning, motivation, and behavior.

Most of my patients who struggle with cravings can make a
link between how they feel and what they crave but are unable
to understand why or how to overcome the nagging desire to
eat something sweet, salty, or processed. The engraved behavior
is hard to overcome when it involves parts of our brain that
purposely drive the well-developed habits. In this chapter, we will
go behind the scenes and see just how the brain works and why
the drive is so powerful.

Since the 1930s, when researchers first started studying
addiction, our understanding of addiction has evolved. It's no

longer a game of will power. Today addiction is recognized as a chronic disease that changes brain structure and function. Just as cardiovascular disease damages the heart, kidneys, and blood vessels, and diabetes impairs the pancreas, addiction damages the brain. This happens as a result of a series of changes that starts with the recognition of the experience of pleasure from an addicting substance, such as a drug or the food drug, sugar, and ends with a drive toward compulsive behavior in order to experience the sensation of pleasure.

In the 1950s, James Olds and Peter Milner implanted electrodes in the brains of rats and allowed the animals to press a lever to receive a mild burst of electrical stimulation to their brains. The two scientists discovered that there were certain areas of the brain that rats would repeatedly press the lever to receive stimulation to. In fact, one of the rats pressed a lever 7500 times over twelve hours to receive electrical stimulation in that particular area of the brain. Eventually, it was recognized that dopamine neurons are activated during this type of rewarding stimulation. Researchers further found that by administrating a drug that blocks the effect of dopamine, they could cause the rats to stop pressing the lever. Without dopamine activity, the rats were less likely to find brain stimulation rewarding.[42]

The brain registers pleasure experienced from sex, drugs, alcohol, money, or a satisfying meal in the same way. This is known as the "pleasure principle," and it affects the brain's reward center. In the brain, the release of the neurotransmitter dopamine is so closely tied to pleasure that neuroscientists refer to the region as the brain's "pleasure center." The pleasure center is made up of two main dopamine travel pathways that are activated by any given reward-producing stimulus. One pathway is located between the ventral tegmental area (VTA) of the brain, a dopamine producing area, and the nucleus accumbens, the motivation and reward center. The second pathway is between the VTA and the cerebral cortex, the most anterior part of the brain that is responsible for key day to day actions like memory, attention, perception, cognition, awareness, language, thought, and, of course, consciousness.

All drugs of abuse, from nicotine to heroin cause a particularly powerful surge of dopamine. The likelihood that using a drug or participating in a rewarding activity like sex or eating a certain food high in sugar and fat will lead to addiction is directly linked to the speed with which it promotes dopamine release, the intensity of that release, and the reliability of that release. One reason food cravings like our desire for sugar and processed foods are so hard to kick is that the intensity and reliability of dopamine release is similar to that of substances like cocaine, alcohol, and nicotine, which target the same pleasure pathways.

Sugar and other substances are addicting not only because of the dopamine surge and the pleasure that follows, but also because dopamine plays a very important role in learning and memory—you taste sugar enough times over the years to learn and remember that it makes you feel good. Dopamine also interacts with a neurotransmitter called glutamate to further solidify the reward-related behavior. It's a perfectly orchestrated dance.

The dopamine-glutamate connection is important because of its role in linking life-sustaining behaviors like sex and eating with pleasure and reward. Addictive substances and behaviors stimulate the same circuit as do the life-sustaining behaviors. Repeated exposure causes nerve cells in the nucleus accumbens and the prefrontal area of the brain involved in planning and executing tasks to communicate in such a way that it couples liking something (sugar) with wanting it. This whole process drives us to act on the want and encourages us to seek out the source of pleasure.[43]

Anyone who has tried to give up sugar or other processed foods has suffered from a hangover that is similar to giving up caffeine, nicotine, or other drugs: headaches, fatigue, irritability, brain fog, depression, and, of course, craving the substance. This occurs because sugar consumption over time changes the brain's reward system. Sugar directly elevates the brain's dopamine levels.

When sugary foods are consumed on a regular basis, the brain thinks it can kick back, relax, and take a break from making its own dopamine.[44] The craving happens when you stop the habit of eating sugar or processed foods, and you experience the dramatic dip in dopamine levels, which makes you feel subpar, to say the least. This classically happens when people embark on a cleanse or a challenge that encourages elimination of processed foods, sugar, and alcohol. Initially, many people experience withdrawal symptoms, but over time as the body adapts, the symptoms subside, and you no longer feel bound to the cravings—a happy place to be. But when the cleanse or challenge is over, most people resort to old eating habits and behaviors, which instantly activates the pleasure pathways. I spend a good chunk of my time with patients, talking about how to turn any nutrition plan into a lifestyle rather than a diet with a starting and ending point. At the end of this book, you will find many solutions to creating change that lasts, but for now, let's continue the journey through the brain. The players involved make it fascinating!

Besides dopamine, the other major neurotransmitters to consider, which are related to cravings, are serotonin, GABA, and acetylcholine. It is common to be depleted in more than one of these neurotransmitters. We briefly talked about serotonin in chapter one when we looked at sugar and its impact on serotonin release. From chapter two, you are familiar with dopamine and its effect on pleasure. In this next section, we take a deeper look at what these neurotransmitters do and the classical symptoms associated with their deficiency. I have yet to find someone who doesn't experience a set of these symptoms to some extent on a daily basis. You're not alone; trust me on this one!

Our metabolism, mood, and energy at any given moment in time is highly dependent on the interaction between these four key neurotransmitters. Dopamine and acetylcholine are known to be stimulating, while neurotransmitters serotonin and GABA are sedating or relaxing to the nervous system and are commonly prescribed as appetite suppressants in the form of

Serotonin Reuptake Inhibitors (SSRI's). As you make your way to the end of this chapter, I'll show you how you can correct a neurotransmitter deficiency naturally—no anti-depressants or appetite suppressants needed.

Although it may seem that your cravings come out of nowhere, there's definitely rhyme and reason for why we experience them. In optimal amounts, dopamine is stimulating, energizing, and motivating. People report feeling as if they are in the zone, have no trouble focusing, and have a high drive to achieve. You can guess what a deficiency of dopamine may look like. Low levels of dopamine can present as inability to focus, low energy, and loss of interest. What do you crave when your energy is low and you're apathetic to the task at hand? Sugar, chocolate, and coffee, of course—the very things that occupy our pantries, office break rooms, and desk drawers. In moderation, consumption of these products can provide a natural dopamine release. But when consumed in excessive amounts, they can lead to excessive dopamine stimulation and, over time, can weaken the natural dopamine release resulting in constant cravings to get the same effect.

The other stimulating brain chemical, acetylcholine, plays a vital role in processing information, problem solving, memory, recollection of people and places, and the brain's ability to fight fatigue. A good example of its deficiency is classically seen in conditions like Alzheimer's disease, where there is severe memory impairment. How is this related to food cravings? Low levels of this neurotransmitter can present with symptoms of forgetfulness, mental fog, and cognitive decline. People can experience strong cravings for fat, because it contains the essential nutrient and building block for acetylcholine called choline. Common junk food cravings associated with its deficiency include fried foods, burgers, and pizza. However, if you're one of the lucky ones who has trained your palette to crave healthy fats, cravings can be for nuts, avocados, and eggs. When I first embarked on my journey to a crave-free life, I loaded on these healthy fats. For every pizza craving, I substituted a healthy fat and carbohydrate. Even while

I was pregnant, I would flip the craving on its back and see it from a different perspective. Was my body really craving the junk food, or was it a sign that I needed more whole foods? Of course, allowing yourself to be human and enjoy a slice of pizza once in a while is definitely part of making it sustainable. But when it comes to changing behavior and developing good habits, you need to focus on filling up with foods that are nutrient dense and support brain health.

I've previously discussed serotonin and its powerful and addicting relationship to sugar. People with low serotonin levels who suffer from depression and low self-esteem and have trouble sleeping complain of craving starchy and salty foods, such as bread and pasta, salty cheese, and pretzels. Lower than normal serotonin levels can also make it challenging to stick to a low carbohydrate diet because of insatiable cravings for carbs and can leave folks cranky, pessimistic, frustrated, and irritable. There are many natural ways to boost serotonin levels. I will cover this in detail along with the other neurotransmitters at the end of this chapter.

The last neurotransmitter is GABA, which is responsible for making us feel relaxed, stress less, and sleep better at night. Normal GABA levels help us manage anxiety and make it easy for us to turn our backs on cravings and the desire to overindulge. Unfortunately, those of us who have lower than normal GABA can experience poor stress management, sleep disturbance, and even symptoms of Irritable Bowel Syndrome. As opposed to other neurotransmitter deficiencies, which manifest in food cravings and mood changes, low GABA levels don't result in a particular craving but instead create a strong desire to consume large amounts of food...quickly. This is relevant in cases of emotional eating where, hungry or not, eating becomes a matter of using food to reach peak emotional state rather than to satisfy an empty stomach.

Given what we know about the function and importance of neurotransmitters on our mood and cravings, there are many reasons why someone may experience their deficiency in the first place.

Neurotransmitters are made from amino acids, which are obtained from protein in our diet. We need vitamins and minerals from our food to help create them as well. A poor diet, such as the Standard American Diet (SAD, so sad), lacks the essential building blocks necessary for optimal brain health.

Furthermore, pharmaceutical medications prescribed to correct neurotransmitter deficiencies can actually cause a depletion of neurotransmitters like serotonin, as seen in treatments for depression with SSRI's. By increasing the brain levels of serotonin with a pharmaceutical agent, the body increases the breakdown of naturally produced serotonin causing the levels to decline, as medications like the SSRI's just recirculate the already low level of the neurotransmitter. The brain's feedback loops register that there's enough serotonin in circulation and down-regulate the production.

Common mood enhancers such as coffee, guarana, and chocolate, particularly when they are paired, provide a short-term fix to an ongoing problem, such as daily fatigue and burnout, but can further reduce the effectiveness of neurotransmitters over time. When we drink coffee, the caffeine impacts brain chemistry by binding to proteins in the brain called adenosine receptors. Used in moderation, which most of us fail to do, caffeine can improve cognitive function and help us with complex tasks at work, at school, or in performance. But one of the reasons we go past one cup of coffee a day is that we quickly build tolerance to caffeine. In order to make up for adenosine receptors that have been inhibited by caffeine, the brain creates more receptors and as a result, more caffeine is needed throughout the day to keep the same level of energy.[46]

Rather than rely on sugary substances and copious amounts of caffeine to compensate for a neurotransmitter deficiency or resort to a pharmaceutical drug like an SSRI, it is possible to naturally correct an imbalance to start feeling your best.

Neurotransmitters, such as serotonin, are synthesized from compounds commonly derived from food. Serotonin is so important in regulating our appetite that it is commonly termed as the brain's satiety chemical, as it has the power to turn our appetite on and off, and most importantly, regulate cravings.

The key to optimal serotonin production and the prevention of food cravings includes increasing serotonin levels before meals and triggering serotonin production before cravings onset and during times of stress, when we want to overeat carbohydrates. *The Serotonin Power Diet* by Dr. Wurtman and Dr. Frusztajer talks about just that, utilizing over thirty years of research to show how eating certain types of carbohydrates can help boost serotonin production, improve mood, diminish cravings, and liberate you from the common appetite suppressants prescribed to lose weight.

Snacks are the most important part of boosting serotonin. The types of snacks and the timing of snacks affect the amount of serotonin produced by your brain and influence how well you maintain those levels throughout the day. The ability to regulate our cravings by regulating serotonin levels goes to show that it's not all about willpower—there is reason and science behind cravings. The trick to eating carbohydrates to boost optimal levels of serotonin is not eat too much or you'll get the obvious opposite effect—weight gain, which may be one of the reasons you're reading this book in the first place.

Please note that this is one of many ways that you can naturally boost the production of serotonin. If this particular method interests you, I recommend that you look into the book by Dr. Wurtman. But for now, here are a few quick tips to get you started.

According to Dr. Wurtman, it's important to eat the carbohydrates on an empty stomach in order avoid interference with protein from a previous meal. To do this, wait about three hours after a meal that contained protein. Although it is recommended to eat a refined carbohydrate like graham crackers or pretzels, because they are easily digested and absorbed and rapidly release serotonin, I've explained the addictive nature of these types of carbohydrates earlier. I recommend eating different types of carbohydrates that are also quickly digested but have greater nutritional value. Ideally, the serving should contain twenty-five to thirty-five grams of carbohydrates and no more than four grams of protein and three grams of fat to prevent the slowing of digestion.[47] Think of foods like banana, whole grain crackers, sweet potato, or plain oatmeal to get started.

This is one of many ways you can naturally increase serotonin levels. I am about to show how you can naturally support production of other neurotransmitters by tuning in to what the body is trying to tell you. Balancing things naturally is always the first best course of action before resorting to something more serious and potentially harmful, which is the case with pharmaceutical drugs. Because neurotransmitters are synthesized from amino acid precursors (think protein), it is easy to supplement or eat foods that contain some of these building blocks.

Put this chapter into action by following the exercise provided, along with the action steps to balance neurotransmitters naturally for fewer cravings, increased mental focus, and better daily performance.

► **CHAPTER 3 EXERCISE:** Which Neurotransmitters Are Involved?

Use the questionnaire below to help identify which neurotransmitters you may be deficient in. This is not meant to be a medical diagnosis but a tool you can use to better understand the reasons behind your cravings, feelings, and mood. Once you complete the questionnaire, you can follow the suggestions for food and supplements that can naturally alter the production of the specific neurotransmitters.

For this purpose, I have also designed a product, **Crave Reset, Ultimate Craving Control**, which you can get by going to **sproactivehealthnd.com/shopwellness** to specifically target neurotransmitter deficiencies and help improve mood, manage stress, and decrease the need to reach for something sweet, salty, or crunchy. Given the combination of neurotransmitter precursors, vitamins, and herbs, the **Crave Reset** formula is an all-natural and effective way to regain control of your mental and physical health.

Is Serotonin Deficiency a Problem? Add up the points and see!

1. Do you tend to have negative or pessimistic thoughts? 3 pt.
2. Do you find yourself often worried or anxious with difficulty staying in the present? *3 pt.*
3. Are you troubled with low self-esteem or lack of self-confidence? *3 pt.*
4. Do you frequently experience irritability, anger bursts, mood fluctuations, or depressed mood? *2 pt.*
5. Do you routinely like to have sweet or starchy snacks, wine, tobacco, marijuana, or other recreational drugs? *3 pt.*
6. Are you a light sleeper or someone who has restless sleep? *2 pt.*
7. Have you ever had unexplained muscle pain, such as with Fibromyalgia or other similar symptoms? *3 pt.*
8. Have you had fibromyalgia (unexplained muscle pain) or TMJ (pain, tension, and grinding associated with your jaw)? *3 pt.*

If your score adds up to more than 10, chances are you have low serotonin levels.

Things That Can Help Serotonin Deficiency:

Supplementing with serotonin amino acid precursors, such as tryptophan, 5-HTP, or SAM-e, can be highly beneficial. You may also find that including tryptophan-rich foods like raw cacao, turkey, pork, duck, and chicken can help you kick the sugar habit, reduce cravings, and minimize highs and lows in mood.

Consider also supplementing with my highly effective **Crave Reset**, formula for best results!

Feeling down and motivated by food?
The next set of questions identifies Dopamine Deficiencies!

1. Do you find yourself often depressed or feeling flat? *3 pt.*
2. Is your stress threshold, energy, and mental focus low? *2 pt.*
3. Do you have trouble focusing or have you been prescribed Attention Deficit Disorder medication? *2 pt.*
4. Do you experience low drive, motivation, or inability to experience pleasure from life? *2 pt.*
5. Do you feel that in order to be motivated or energized, you need coffee, sugar, energy drinks, or other substances? *3 pt.*
6. Do you easily put on weight? *2 pt.*
7. Are you an adrenaline junkie or a risk taker? *3 pt.*
8. Are you affected by cold easily? *2 pt.*

If your score adds up to more than 10, chances are you have low dopamine levels.

Things that can help Dopamine Deficiency:

As with serotonin, you can boost dopamine production by consuming protein from lean meats like turkey and also by including raw cocoa in your daily nutrition. You will find plenty of delicious recipes throughout the book that use raw cacao in smoothies and raw treats. Not only do these recipes balance your blood sugar and curb cravings, but they also support healthy brain chemistry! If you need a little extra support, you can also try supplementing with tyrosine, a precursor to dopamine, which is also found in my **Crave Reset.**

Feeling stressed or overworked, and reaching for a snack to help feel happy and manage stress? The next set of questions are about identifying a GABA Deficiency!

1. Do you always feel under pressure or suffer from self-imposed deadlines? *3 pt.*

2. Are you irritated, frustrated, or upset when stressed? *2 pt.*
3. Do you feel overwhelmed? *3 pt.*
4. Do you experience feeling of shakiness or weakness when under stress? *2 pt.*
5. Is there a history of panic attacks? *3 pt.*
6. Are you sensitive to light, sound, or smell? *3 pt.*
7. Do you have a hard time skipping meals? *3 pt.*
8. Do you use food to calm down? *2 pt.*

If your score adds up to more than 10, chances are you have low GABA levels.

Things that can help GABA Deficiency:

With a GABA deficiency, reach for food items like shell fish, broccoli, brown rice, and bananas. These contain high amounts of GABA amino acid precursors – such as L-Glutamine, Theanine, Leucine, and Taurien— all necessary to create GABA. However, if you still find yourself overly stressed and pressured and have the tendency to use food for comfort, then try supplementing with a GABA supplement.

Feeling slow or sluggish? Answer the following questions to see if low Acetylcholine levels are to blame!

1. Do you feel as if you experience mental fog on a regular basis? *3 pt.*
2. Have you noticed a cognitive decline? *2 pt.*
3. Do you have trouble with recollection and memory in general? *3 pt.*
4. Do you frequently experience dry eyes and mouth? *3 pt.*
5. Have you suffered from inflammatory or autoimmune conditions, such as Multiple Sclerosis? *2 pt.*
6. Is your libido low? *2 pt.*
7. Do you find yourself scrambling to find the right words or have difficulty speaking? *2 pt.*
8. Do you have strong cravings for fat? *3 pt.*

If your score adds up to more than 10, chances are you have low acetylcholine levels.

Things that can help Acetylcholine Deficiency:

For low acetylcholine production, reach for food sources that contain plenty of healthy fats, such as eggs, olives, nuts, avocados, fish, and coconut oil. These are great alternatives to the common high fat and processed foods that people tend to reach for. Turn to the back of the book for recipes and mood-enhancing snack ideas that are packed with healthy fats! You can also try supplementing with the acetylcholine precursor lecithin in the form of a nutrient called phosphatidylcholine.

CHAPTER 4:
Nutrition and Nutrient Deficiencies—The Link

"Is there really one 'right way' to eat for all people with diverse ethnic heritages and modified DNA? Are we making foods culprits rather than examining what the environment has done to the food?"

—DEANNA MINICH, PH.D., FUNCTIONAL MEDICINE NUTRITIONIST

AND RESEARCHER AT FOOD & SPIRIT

There are a lot of opinions circulating concerning the best way to eat. Foods get put on banned lists, and people have panic attacks over it, because they find out that certain foods they've been eating are "bad" based on someone else's poor research. Various diets promote a high fat, low carb, and high protein way of eating that is hard to sustain, not really environmentally friendly, and works for some and not for others. There are great benefits to those diets, but they're not for everyone. I have found that there is a lot of confusion regarding how much protein is safe to consume, what are good fats versus bad fats, and how much coconut oil one should really eat when it's in everything these days.

The bottom line to eating a specific way for a certain amount of time is that it becomes limiting—nutritionally and psychologically. As a quick example, some popular dietary recommendations limit the intake of legumes and grains because of a compound called phytic acid that is found in this food group. Because phytic acid binds to key nutrients like iron, zinc, and magnesium and can prevent their absorption, it has gotten massive attention. But most research studies show that phytic acid actually has beneficial properties and that eating a diverse diet is one of the best ways to prevent a nutritional deficiency.

I have clients who do exceptionally well on a vegan diet with the bulk of their nutrition coming from lentils, beans, grains, fermented soy produce, veggies, and fruits. But I also have clients who do very poorly on such a diet and rely on meat for most of their sources of protein. I have also had clients who decided to jump from a mostly paleo diet to a vegan diet only to have their bodies scream at them with all sorts of gut upset, mood swings, and, of course, cravings.

Nutrition is very personal, and how the body responds to any nutritional change is also very individualistic based on metabolism, genetics, activity level, stress, and physiologic make up. Food cravings, along with other symptoms, can be a major sign that something is missing from the diet. Instead of resisting it, addressing it with the right nutrition and supplements can make a difference between short-term and long-term success.

One of my patients came to see me one morning and thanked me for "giving back" her breakfast smoothie, which had been her go-to in the mornings but was considered a banned item in the diet she was following. She mentioned that her mornings were so much better, and her kids and husband were happy about it too. The diet my patient was on stated that re-creating baked goods, junk foods, or treats with approved ingredients was not allowed and might not be psychologically healthy. My patient considered her smoothie, which had pea protein (a "banned" ingredient), blueberries, spinach, cashews, and unsweetened almond milk to be a treat after she read the dietary guidelines. She said, "It provided a little bit of sweetness and the perfect amount of protein and fat for me and was my go-to most mornings. But with the diet, I felt like I couldn't have something like it, because it would be considered a treat—even a healthy treat."

Any diet can leave an imprint on a person's psyche and physiology in the form nutrient deficiencies and hormone imbalances as you'll see in future chapters. Don't get me wrong, most of these diets are superior to the Standard American Diet, but they can still leave people feeling deprived and malnourished, and can lead to poor health outcomes (elevated cardiovascular disease markers as an example) for multiple reasons, including being restrictive in some ways (such as very few carbs) or overly abundant in others (such as lots of protein and fat).

Food groups that have been attacked by popular dietary trends and called poison include grains, legumes, and dairy. Most of these foods are overly processed and nutrient depleted today, and we've developed food sensitivities towards them. But not all grains, legumes, and dairy are created equal, and having them on a banned list can certainly affect our nutrient landscape and balance. I've had patients who experienced fatigue and slow digestion without grains, only to regain vitality and improved digestion after introducing grains back into their diet. Some of my clients who were on a restrictive low carbohydrate diet felt irritable, craved sugar, and had severe mental fog. One of the things I did was provide education: not all grains are created equal. Not all grains contain gluten, wheat-free does not mean gluten-free, not everyone is wheat or gluten sensitive, and there are many gluten-free grains. I also spent a lot of time talking about the difference between various carbohydrates found in different foods. A sweet potato is not nutritionally the same as a potato, for example.

The reason I talk about grains in particular is because, from my professional observation, I've seen that grains are the main focus of elimination with most dietary trends. Food cravings can be a result of swinging to the extreme sides of the pendulum. Too many carbohydrates from the wrong source, and you are hooked on sugar and processed foods. Too few good quality carbohydrates from nutrient dense foods, and you feel awful.

Working with a diverse patient base, I have observed that in most cultures, grains and legumes are a staple. Only recently have certain dietary trends identified them as bad for all the wrong reasons. Sure, if you strip away the essential nutrients of a food to the point of no recognition, then over time that will cause distress in the body, which is what we've seen happen with Celiac, Crohn's, and other conditions, such as IBS and Leaky Gut Syndrome. Gluten-containing grains, including wheat, have given other grains a bad reputation.

The takeaway message here is that what the popular diets have in common is that they are not sustainable in the long run given their restrictive nature. They will have you running for the fridge when willpower stops working. In my clinical practice, I frequently hear people say, "It worked for a month, but then I couldn't stick with it, and then different foods started to sneak back in, as did the weight." There are a number of ways to make any diet more sustainable, but this is the most important piece of the puzzle that people are missing. Understanding what nutrients are missing from your current diet, learning how to replenish them in the best way possible, and knowing the best food combinations to increase satiety and decrease food cravings are extremely important to making any diet work, whether you are struggling to eat clean or are on the right track already.

Nutrient deficiencies is one of the main reasons I stay away from any diet that bans grains or legumes, as you'll read in a moment. In later chapters, where I discuss food sensitivities and elimination, I'll talk about eliminating foods and reintroducing them. If you are sensitive to these foods, then, of course, staying away from them will prove to be more beneficial than not. But if you have no food sensitivity to certain grains or legumes, then not having them just because a certain diet program tells you not to is not a good reason.

Consider, too, that there is yet another major reason why some people have a harder time sticking to any particular diet while others don't. Research has shown that people's metabolism for carbohydrates, protein, and fat varies. The different physiological and biochemical processes in the body, such as glucose metabolism in the liver, production and release of insulin, fat storage and breakdown, and appetite control, are dependent on our genetic predisposition.[11] In addition, the "Current Opinion" in *Clinical Nutrition and Metabolic Care* has found that expression of certain genes, such as the ones that regulate fatty acid metabolism, are related to certain diseases as well as our overall metabolism.[12] Health is not as easy as following any certain diet. Many variables should be considered. A more individualistic approach to any nutrition program is necessary for the best health outcomes and results.

There are many examples of nutrient deficiencies we can look at to see what's behind the common sweet, salty, and fatty food cravings. My patient who adored her morning smoothie was a very active and overall healthy female who frequently did all sorts of dietary challenges, took the best supplements, and was very well educated in the realm of nutrition. No matter what she did, though, she could not let go of the tortilla chips. She described her craving for the salty and crunchy with such a delight and spark in her eyes that I knew we needed to look deeper.

The following recommendations for nutrient deficiencies and their respective cravings are adapted from the book *Choose Your Foods: Like Your Life Depends on Them,* by Dr. Colleen Huber.[31]

CHOCOLATE

If you crave chocolate, the most likely culprit is a deficiency in magnesium. I experienced this personally after giving birth to our first child. I was putting cocoa in everything, including smoothies and oatmeal, and I was eating chocolate like crackers. Taking a good magnesium supplement can help tremendously (in the absence of any other underlying health conditions, of course), and loading up on magnesium rich foods, such as raw nuts, seeds, legumes, and fruit, can help.

SWEETS

Chromium, carbon, phosphorous, sulfur, and tryptophan deficiencies can lead to the cravings of sweets. Foods rich in chromium include broccoli, grapes, cheese, dried beans, and chicken. Fresh fruits are rich in carbon. Foods like eggs, fish, nuts, legumes, dairy, and grains have plenty of phosphorous. Cruciferous vegetables, such as kale and cabbage, contain sulfur. Lastly, if you're looking to increase your tryptophan levels, consider adding more lamb, raisins, sweet potatoes, and spinach to your diet.

FATTY FOODS

If your cravings are more for oily or fatty foods, then consider a calcium deficiency. Of course, a calcium deficiency together with other bone-building nutrients, such as Magnesium, Zinc, Vitamin K, and Vitamin D, can manifest itself in other ways, but craving fatty foods is one of many. Food rich in calcium (note, no dairy!) include mustard greens, root vegetables like turnips, broccoli, kale, and legumes.

SALTY FOODS

When it comes to cravings for salty foods, chloride is a very important mineral to look into. It is common to be deficient in chloride, because chloride is lost through perspiration, such as sweating during exercise and overusing coffee and other diuretics, including pharmaceutical drugs. Preventing an overall mineral deficiency can be accomplished by consuming water with electrolytes and foods rich in chloride, such as raw goat milk, fish, and unrefined sea salt. Back to my patient who had a serious tortilla chip problem: She worked out five to six days a week, ate a very high protein diet, and was limiting the amount of sodium she consumed, based on recommendations from her other healthcare provider. Diversifying her protein sources to include more fish and less meat and using sea salt in moderation during cooking helped her get the serious salt craving under control.

The best way to find out how deficient you are in particular nutrients is to do a blood test. There are specific labs that specialize in just that and can provide a comprehensive nutrient analysis that can tell you everything from what you're missing to how well your immune system is functioning based on the nutrients available. The test I use in my practice is called **SpectraCell Micronutrient Test Analysis.** If you go on the company's webpage, you can order a kit and also find a provider who can go over the results with you. It is one of my favorite comprehensive tests that anyone can do. When you do a lab test, know that it reflects your past six months. That means that loading up on fruits, vegetables, and berries and eating a whole-foods diet a week before the test won't improve your results!

Once you know what you are deficient in, the next step is to replenish from inside out. This includes following a diet rich in the nutrients you need and also including supplements to help expedite the replenishment process. Keep in mind that how well your body is able to bounce back from a nutrient deficiency is dependent on the function of your digestive system or your gut. Years ago, I heard a physiology professor say, "You are not just what you eat. You are what you absorb." If your gut function is not optimal for whatever reason, then taking good supplements and eating the right foods may not do much. In fact, having the cleanest diet may not make a difference either if your gut function is not great.

The next chapter covers just that: the importance of our gut on our mood, feelings and cravings, and how to keep it healthy so it can work for us rather than against us. I will show how eating specific foods and taking supplements that are gut protective, nourishing, and restorative can make a world of a difference in correcting nutrient deficiencies and preventing them from happening in the long run.

Before moving on to the next chapter, take a moment to look through the tips and suggestions listed at the end of this chapter to help you get through the gnarliest of cravings, whether you are cutting out sugar, decreasing carb intake, or putting yourself through a clean eating challenge!

➤CHAPTER 4 EXERCISES: Finding the Right Food
Best Food Combinations and Alternatives For
Optimal Health, Energy, and Vitality

You guys are in for a treat here! I LOVE this section, as it provides you with fail- proof food combinations that can literally be used to rescue you from the 'hangry' stage of the day. I am also providing you with some tasty food alternatives to the typical sugary, salty, and fatty snacks that many of us crave! Enjoy.

BEST FOOD COMBINATIONS TO BEAT THE HANGRY:

The best way to keep your energy and mood stable is to maintain blood sugar levels, balanced by having smaller meals throughout the day. There's a time and a place to have carbohydrates alone, such as when you're trying the serotonin boosting diet, or you want to have carbs pre- or post-workout for energy and recovery, but those situations aside, I recommend pairing carb rich foods with a source of fat or protein. This pairing slows digestion, decreases the rate at which blood sugar spikes and dips, and creates a more stable internal environment.

The following snack suggestions are best consumed between meals when you feel like reaching for a sugary snack, you're drawn to the vending machine, or you're running on empty and it's still awhile before meal time:

- Apple or banana with cashew or almond butter
- Celery sticks and hummus
- Cucumber slices with avocado, drizzled with olive oil, and Himalayan sea salt (I use this instead of crackers!)
- Cucumber slices with salsa and/or hummus (I eat this instead of chips and dip.)

- 1/2 cups of nuts with 1/2 cup of berries and dairy-free yogurt
- Avocado and tomato slices with basil, olive oil, and apple cider vinegar instead of balsamic (I love this as an alternative to the caprese salad!)
- Turkey lettuce wraps with or without avocado (This has been a life saver for me. When I am on the go and need to have quick snack with me, this is one of my go-to's.) You can add cucumbers to this, spice it up, dress it up with truffle oil and a splash of balsamic vinegar, or keep it simple! A vegan/vegetarian option is chickpeas or cooked lentils, which is also a great and tasty option.

ALTERNATIVES FOR SUGARY, SALTY, AND FATTY FOOD CRAVINGS:

My recommendation is that you not only use these recipes for their nourishing properties but also use them when you want to indulge guilt-free while knowing you're doing something good for the body. All my recipes are SUPER easy to make and require very little time. I've used them over the years for desserts and snacks or simply when I'm running out of the house!

SWEET TOOTH MENDERS:

Here are a few sweet suggestions for the times you crave cake, candy, ice cream, and anything that gets your sweet tooth going. I was able to overcome some of my hard-to-beat sugar cravings years back when I started on this path, and I can personally attest that some of these suggestions have helped me outgrow my need for sugar, carbs, and processed foods.

Creamy Coconut Cashew Smoothie with optional add ons

Makes 1 smoothie

1 cup coconut water

1/3 cup raw cashews or 2 tablespoons of cashew butter

1 fresh or frozen banana

1 pitted date

A dash of cinnamon and Himalayan Salt

Optional add-ons: spirulina, flax seeds, raw cacao, mint, and pea or rice protein.

Place all of the ingredients into your blender and blend on high until the desired consistency is reached.

Matcha Green Tea Fudge Bites
Makes about 20-24 pieces

1 cup coconut butter

1/3 cup cream from canned coconut milk (adding the liquid portion of the coconut milk will make the fudge separate)

3 Tbsp coconut oil

2 Tbsp matcha green tea powder

2 tsp vanilla extract

1/2 cup maple syrup or honey

Optional Himalayan Sea Salt to taste

1/2 cup of toasted, shredded coconut.

While melting the coconut butter and coconut oil in a small saucepan over low-medium heat, whisk in the coconut cream. Add the matcha green tea, vanilla, maple syrup, and the optional sea salt, while making sure everything blends well. Taste as you go – this is the best part!

Spoon the mixture into parchment paper-lined 6x8" pan or something similar. Sprinkle with the toasted, shredded coconut, and let it cool in the refrigerator for a few hours.

Cut into desired pieces and enjoy!

Super Power Cookies—and super tasty too!
Makes 12 cookies

You can freeze these and thaw them out as needed, which is very convenient for the days that you're on the go and need a quick breakfast or snack.

1 medium banana, mashed

8 medjool dates

1/2 cup walnuts

1/2 cup ground flax seed or chia seeds

1/2 cup pumpkin seeds or sunflower seeds

1/2 cup raisins

1/4 goji berries

3 tablespoons hemp seeds

2 tablespoons of cacao nibs

1 cup shredded coconut

water if needed

Preheat oven to 300°F. Puree the dates and banana in a food processor. Move the mixture into a large bowl and mix in all the other ingredients. At this point you can add some water if the mixture seems too dry. Roll pieces of mixture into balls, place on a cookie sheet, and push down with the palm of your hand to flatten. They should be about ½-inch thick. Bake for 25 minutes or until cookies start to color round the edges. Cool to room temperature. Store in the refrigerator for up to a week or freeze.

SALTY SNACK TAMERS:

The snacks below are great for times when you're craving something salty and crunchy.

They are a perfect alternative to chips and crackers and are much friendlier to the waistline. I do recommend making a little more, just because these snacks tend to disappear among friends and family!

Savory Kale Chips
Makes about 2 cups

The nutritional yeast adds a nice cheesy flavor, and salt paired with a crunch hits the spot! Feel free to leave out any of the spices or add ones that you prefer if you're looking for a specific flavor.

1 bunch kale leaves

1 tablespoon extra-virgin olive oil or melted coconut oil

1.5-2 tablespoons nutritional yeast

1.5 teaspoon garlic powder

3/4 teaspoon chili powder

1 tsp teaspoon onion powder

3/4 teaspoon smoked paprika

1/4 teaspoon fine grain sea salt or pink Himalayan sea salt

1/8 teaspoon cayenne pepper (optional)

Preheat oven to 300°F and line a large, rimmed baking sheet with parchment paper. Remove leaves from the stems of the kale and roughly tear it up into large pieces. Wash and dry and place in a large bowl. Massage the kale in olive oil or coconut oil and add the spices to combine. Place seasoned kale onto the baking sheet and make sure that it forms a single layer. Bake for 25 mins, rotating the baking sheet occasionally. Cool kale, and enjoy before the crowd gets to them!

Crispy'n Salty Chickpeas
Makes 2 cups

These delicious chickpeas can be used as a snack or used on top of salads and soups.

Eat them quickly or they become chewy, which is not so bad either!

2 15-oz cans chickpeas

2 Tbsps olive oil or other herbal infused oils that you like, such as
   garlic olive oil

1/2 to 3/4 tsp salt depending on how salty you want them

2 to 4 tsps spices of choice, such as chili powder, curry powder,
   garam masala, cumin, smoked paprika, parsley, or dill.

Heat the oven to 400°F and place an oven rack in the middle of the oven. Rinse and drain the chickpeas: Open the cans of chickpeas, pour them into a strainer in the sink, and rinse them thoroughly under cool running water. Dry the chickpeas by patting with a clean dishtowel or paper towels. You can also let them air dry for a few minutes. Coat the chickpeas with olive oil and salt and spread them out on the baking sheet. You can also use a spatula to stir the chickpeas and make sure they are evenly coated for the best crispy effect. Bake the chickpeas in the oven for 20 to 30 minutes depending on your oven, and stir or shake them about every minutes. They are done when they are golden and slightly darkened, dry and crispy on the outside and soft in the middle—yum!! Last and final step is to toss them with the spices. Ding!

Better Than Potato Chips, Zucchini Chips!
Makes about 50 chips, depending on slicer

1 large zucchini

2 tbsp olive oil or melted coconut oil

Sea salt

Cracked pepper, optional

Preheat oven to 225°F. Line two large baking sheets with parchment paper. Slice your zucchini on a mandolin. The mandolin that I have has settings 1, 2, or 3 for thickness. I used 2 for this recipe. Place the slices of zucchini between two sheets of paper towels and press out any liquid. Line up the zucchini slices on the prepared baking sheet, making sure they do not overlap. Using a pastry brush, coat the slices with the olive oil and then sprinkle with the sea salts and optional cracked pepper. It's best to do a light sprinkle of salt initially and then after the slices are done baking to prevent over-salting. Bake for 2 hours until slices are crisp. Allow to cool and keep in an airtight container for up to 3 days.

FATTY SNACK ALTERNATIVES:

Fatty snack alternatives can be paired with salty snacks for the days when you're really struggling. What you'll notice is that once you make these recipes your staples, over time you won't even crave as much of the processed foods. In fact, the more you incorporate real food dressed up with wholesome ingredients, the less you'll crave, period!

Avolicious Dip
Makes about 1 1/2 cups

This is one of my favorites for so many reasons! It is so versatile. I use this as a dip with zucchini chips, as a spread in veggies wraps, mixed with salads instead of dressing, on top of quinoa bowls, or simply straight up!

3 to 4 oz baby spinach

1 large avocado, peeled and diced

1/3 cup tahini

2 Tbsp fresh lemon juice or lime juice

2 Tbsp of chopped shallot

1/2 tsp ground cumin

2 Tbsp finely chopped cilantro

1/2 tsp sea salt

1/4 cup water

Rinse the spinach and cook until just wilted. Place the spinach with the rest of the ingredients in a food processor and, using the s-blade, process until smooth. Add a little water as needed to get the desired consistency. Serve with your choice of veggies or the delicious zucchini chips listed above!

Nuts So Ordinary Trail Mix:

Makes about 3 cups

I love nuts, especially when they are paired with other ingredients, because they make a perfect snack, provide a great source of fat, and help support good mood, brain function, and tame cravings! I'm such a fan of this recipe that it travels with me in my purse, gym bag, car, plane, and stroller and follows me anywhere I go. Next time you're craving that fat slice of pizza, grab a handful of this trail mix, take a moment to enjoy the goodness it provides, relax, and let your craving pass you by. When I was pregnant, pizza was something I could have eaten every day. I didn't. Instead, I found healthy fat and carb alternatives to help me get the nutrition I was craving in healthy ways.

Mix:

1/2 cup almonds

1/2 cup cashews

1/2 cup walnuts

1/2 cup goji berries

1/2 cup cacao nibs

1/2 cup pumpkin seeds

1/2 cup toasted coconut chips

I recommend raw nuts, as they will have the freshest oils, but if you only have access to roasted nuts, that's fine too! I'll take roasted nuts over candy any day. Store in a container in the fridge to optimize freshness.

Power Bowl—You May Feel Like a Super Hero

Makes 1 smoothie bowl. You may want to make a second one later.

This hearty, tasty, satisfying, and hunger-quenching smoothie bowl has a special place in my heart. I've had a lot of great "firsts" in my life. My first great hike, my first trail marathon, my first summit, my first time leading a climb, and my first yoga class, to name just a few. And I can't leave out the first time I met my husband and the first time I saw our baby boy. But when it comes to the journey of food, this one takes the prize. In my personal battle with sugar, recipes like these saved me from the dark side of cravings and helped turn me into a holistic foodie. Spirulina is a superfood. Its properties are magical. This blue-green algae is available in both powders and supplement form and is full of healthy omega-3s like EPA and DHA. This means less inflammation and also less belly fat around the waist! Both pluses. Spirulina is loaded with protein and also contains naturally occurring probiotics.

1 frozen banana

1/2 cup sliced cucumber, skin on or skinless

3/4 - 1 cup coconut milk (I like to get the canned kind, as it is
    creamier and has more healthy fats!)

1 cup frozen spinach

2 tsp spirulina powder

1 Tbsp hemp seed

2 Tbsp protein powder of choice, such as pea, brown rice protein,
    or whey

1/4 cup fresh blueberries

1/4 cup granola, optional

Place all the ingredients in a blender except for the blueberries and granola. Blend until creamy and smooth, adding water or more coconut milk as needed if it's too thick. If it's too thin, add a couple of ice cubes. You want this to be thicker than a smoothie. Scoop into a bowl, and top with blueberries and optional granola. Enjoy before it melts! You can make more and freeze the rest for up to one week.

CHAPTER 5:
It's Not All in Your Head: The Role of Gut Bacteria on Cravings

If you've ever "gone with your gut" to make a decision or felt "butterflies in your stomach" when nervous, you're likely getting signals from an unexpected source: your second brain. Hidden in the walls of the digestive system, this "brain in your gut" is revolutionizing medicine's understanding of the links between digestion, mood, health and even the way you think."

—JOHN HOPKINS MEDICINE, MEDICAL EXPERT

The link between our brain, gut, emotions, and food cravings is undeniable. There are over 100 million nerve cells lining the gastrointestinal system and over 100 trillion bacteria, almost three pounds, that line your intestinal tract! Our digestive tract is a highly complex system that works beyond breaking food down and making it readily available for absorption. Given its complex role, the gut has received a lot of attention in the medical community, as its many processes are linked to mental health, mood, autoimmune disease, endocrine issues, weight loss/weight gain, our general well-being, and, of course, food cravings.

According to a publication in *Nature Reviews Neuroscience*, "Recent neurobiological insights into this gut–brain crosstalk have revealed a complex, bidirectional communication system that not only ensures the proper maintenance of gastrointestinal homeostasis and digestion but is also likely to have multiple effects on affect, motivation and higher cognitive functions, including intuitive decision-making. Moreover, disturbances of this system have been implicated in a wide range of disorders, including functional and inflammatory gastrointestinal disorders, obesity and eating disorders."[13]

A long-time patient of mine didn't realize how dependent she was on sugar and carbohydrates until she actually tried to give them up along with alcohol as part of her New Year resolutions. She and I have worked closely together over the years, but she never brought up any concerns regarding sugar until this moment. Out of curiosity, we decided to do a comprehensive test that looks at all aspects of digestion, including the bacteria. As expected, the bacteria in her gut were having a little party, and she was not invited!

The trillions of bacteria that occupy the gut space are responsible for the secretion of hormones and the neurotransmitters that are then responsible for how we feel, the quality of digestion, appetite and satiety, and even gene expression. If you are not convinced that having a healthy gut can help you feel and look better and can help you understand your cravings better, keep reading. There's more!

Recent research published in *BioEssays* highlights this concept perfectly: "The struggle to resist cravings for foods that are high in sugar and fat is part of daily life for many people. Unhealthy eating is a major contributor to health problems including obesity as well as sleep apnea, diabetes, heart disease, and cancer. Despite negative effects on health and survival, unhealthy eating patterns are often difficult to change. The resistance to change is frequently framed as a matter of 'self-control,' and it has been suggested that multiple 'selves' or cognitive modules exist each vying for control over our eating behavior. Here, we suggest another possibility: that evolutionary conflict between host and microbes in the gut leads microbes to divergent interests over host eating behavior."[16]

So it's not just mind over body. Logically, you may want to make certain dietary changes—like my patient who wanted to give up sugars and alcohol. Realistically, there are many obstacles that need to be overcome to make those changes. One of those obstacles resides within you. The big influence that gut bacteria have on food cravings may explain why it can be so hard to resist and stay away from certain foods—it is almost like having no self-control or facing something beyond your willpower. The gut bacteria that inhabit your gut is a reflection of your current and previous eating habits, among others things, which we will get into soon. It doesn't just happen overnight; rather it is our consistent behavior patterns and food choices that shape our internal landscape over the years.

Different types of bacteria proliferate in the colon based on the different types protein, fat, and carbohydrates we consume on a daily basis. The same research article includes great examples of how different bacteria grow, based on the nutrient composition of the diet. For example, bifidobacteria thrives from a diet high in dietary fiber, while bacteroidetes bacteria has a preference for specific fats. In addition, people can have a different microbiome presentation, depending on where they are from. Specific bacteria that digest seaweed have been identified in people from Japan, while children in Africa, who are raised on sorghum, have unique microbiome that helps to digest the cellulose from the grain. Most importantly, the article mentions that these different bacteria compete with one another. The strongest (or most well-fed) bacteria will win.

The natural conclusion is that cravings for certain foods are heavily dependent on current gut health and the type of bacteria that dominates, which impact the choices we make at our next meal. But more importantly, we can conclude that choosing to eat something other than foods that are processed, refined, or loaded with sugar and sodium will alter the type of bacteria we choose to fuel and help proliferate. That is powerful, because it puts you back in control of your nutrition, and the choices you make regarding your health.

Because of the vital role that our gut bacteria play in our health, including nutrient metabolism and absorption, it's important to first understand what factors affect gut bacteria and how we can support a healthy bacteria population for better mental, emotional, and physical health. Dr. Leo Galland says it best. "We are humans, yes, but we are really ecological systems. The real importance of this in the future of medicine is the recognition that it may be possible to treat people and treat illness by addressing the ecology of the human being rather than just attempting to suppress the disease."

Extensive research has shown that the key factors influencing the growth and development of the gut bacteria include: vaginal or cesarian birth, breastmilk or formula fed during infancy, history of antibiotic use, and the type of diet followed, such as vegan or meat based.[14] In addition, more research suggests that the consumption of carbohydrates, and a specific type of carbohydrate compared to protein and fat, has a direct impact on the bacteria population in our gut including its diversity and proliferation.[8, 15]

Since you picked up this book, chances are you experience some sort of discomfort in your gut or cravings, one way or another. Before good bacteria can repopulate and thrive (so you can do the same), you need to create an optimal internal environment. You start to do that by changing your diet toward eating more anti-inflammatory foods, which happen to promote a healthy gut bacteria population.

The most common foods that have been known to cause inflammation in the gut and have been linked to poor gut health include soy, dairy, gluten, corn, citrus, beef, shellfish, processed foods, peanuts, nightshade vegetables (tomatoes, peppers, eggplant, and potatoes), alcohol, caffeine, and condiments like ketchup, which usually contain preservatives and many additives. However, it's important to realize that even though these foods have been identified as common sources of inflammation, it is very individual-based, and you may have other food sensitivities (not necessarily these) that are causing unnecessary inflammation.

Sugar and processed foods, the very items we develop cravings for, are responsible for a significant amount of gut distress and inflammation. In one study, a professor of genetic epidemiology at King's College London, Tim Spector, wanted to find out what happens to your gut if you eat only fast food. The results of this 10-day trial of eating only fast food were shattering. Almost 40% of his gut bacteria species were lost, which is equivalent to approximately 1,400 different types.[21]

In a recent review published in the *Nutrition Journal,* Dr. Ian Myle explained that today's Westernized diet is setting the stage for a host of immune-mediated chronic diseases.[22] "While today's modern diet may provide beneficial protection from micro and macronutrient deficiencies, our over abundance of calories and the macronutrients that compose our diet may all lead to increased inflammation, reduced control of infection, increased rates of cancer, and increased risk for allergic and auto-inflammatory disease."

Dietary components can either trigger or prevent inflammation, which is responsible for diseases like diabetes, heart disease, stroke, cancer, and much more. The conclusion we arrive at is that consuming high quantities of synthetic trans fats and sugar will increase inflammation, while eating healthy fats, such as omega-3 fats found in fish oil, will help to reduce inflammation. Naturally, the first step to better health becomes identifying and eliminating inflammatory foods. The next step is to provide the body with the building blocks necessary to help keep the gut healthy. There are certain foods and supplements that, when consumed on a regular basis, help the gut function normally, can restore gut lining, and help the proliferation of good gut bacteria.

Foods high in fiber, such as leafy greens, gluten free grains like quinoa, and fruit, not only will keep your bowel movements more regular but will also help you fuel good bacteria by being a great source of fructooligosaccharides or FOS, a by-product from the digestion of fiber-rich foods. Although FOS is available in a supplement form, you get plenty from consuming plant foods like bananas, artichokes, onion, and asparagus, among many others.[23]

Keeping your diet rich in fermented foods, such as kimchi, pickled ginger, or sauerkraut, is also a great way to keep the gut healthy. Fermented foods contain probiotics that have been known to improve the health of intestinal cells, facilitate proper immune response, and decrease allergies along with inflammation.

These foods directly provide your gut with healthy, live micro-organisms that will push out the unhealthy bacteria and, in turn, improve the absorption of nutrients, while improving overall health.[24]

A word of caution here: If you are having any issues with your digestion, please consult your healthcare provider before starting any new nutrition plan. Although the foods recommended for optimal gut health have great benefits, there are cases where a severe bacterial imbalance, such as with Small Intestinal Bacterial Overgrowth (SIBO), will aggravate symptoms. Correcting the overgrowth would be the first natural step toward laying the foundation for optimal health and applying the principles for overall gut health.

My philosophy is that good food comes first, and supplements come second. However, sometimes food is not enough to help the gut heal, and supplementation becomes the next level of intervention to help the body get to where it can function optimally. There are key nutrients that aid in digestion and absorption and help in keeping the gut lining healthy. These include L-glutamine, magnesium, probiotics, digestive enzymes, and deglycerized licorice root (DGL):

L-GLUTAMINE is an essential amino acid, meaning your body must obtain it from food or a supplement source. It serves multiple functions and supports digestive and brain health, muscle development, and weight loss and improves athletic performance. Research has shown that L-Glutamine has the ability to prevent gut deterioration and permeability, and rebuild gut lining.[25]

MAGNESIUM is available in three different forms. Magnesium glycinate and malate are easily absorbed and are more bioavailable for optimal cell function. Magnesium is often overlooked when it comes to gut health, but it can help relax the smooth and skeletal muscle that make up the GI tract to help with bowel movement and promote elimination.[26] I've had many patients say that when they skip their nightly dose of magnesium, it throws off their digestion for a couple of days!

PROBIOTICS in supplemental form, compared with those derived from the afore-mentioned fermented foods, can be a great way to repopulate good gut bacteria and crowd out trouble-causing bacteria. It is important to get probiotics from both food and supplement sources to get the most variety and because food sources usually contain additional fructooligosaccharides (FOS), mentioned previously, that serve as fuel for the bacteria population. Aim to get at least 50 Billion CFU daily, as anything below that may not have the same effect.[27] You can achieve this by choosing a probiotic that contains this amount in either one or multiple servings.

Which probiotics are better? This is a very popular question with no easy answer. With many brands populating stores, it is hard not to grab a bottle that claims to be effective or superior to other brands. Many studies have been conducted, particularly at UC Davis, looking at different types of bacteria and their efficacy at repopulating the gut microbiome. Unfortunately, not all probiotics are created equal, and most won't make it to the colon intact to serve their purpose. Even if they do, they are greeted with a whole lot of other bacteria that will compete for their spot in the arena—survival is minimal.

This is where a comprehensive digestion test comes in to first evaluate if there is a bacterial imbalance and, if so, what needs to be removed, corrected, and repopulated. In my private practice, I use a test called **GI Effects by Genova Laboratories,** but your healthcare provider may recommend a test that works in a similar way or may be better for you. It can help you get a baseline for your current gut health, and you can repeat the test in the future to evaluate how well a treatment plan is working.

In the case of my patient, when I found out that she had a bacterial imbalance, not necessarily overgrowth, I was able to prescribe dietary guidelines and a specific probiotic along with supplements unique to her situation. After six weeks of being on an anti-inflammatory diet along with the prescribed supplements, my patient noticed a significant difference in her energy, sleep, and, of course, her cravings for sugar. The cookie monster was contained, as she said.

DIGESTIVE ENZYMES help break down fats, protein, and carbohydrates. The better these macronutrients are broken down, the better the absorption and utilization of nutrients. Most people with food sensitivities show signs of poorly digested food. Digestive enzymes ensure that food is fully digested and that partially undigested food does not damage the gut wall and cause unnecessary inflammation.[28] Common digestive enzymes include amylase to help with carbohydrate breakdown, protease to aid with protein digestion, and lipase, which helps utilize fat. Amylase is heavily at work when you first start chewing your food, so slowing down at meal time can improve digestion, as the enzyme can do a better job at breaking down the food. The other enzymes kick into gear later in the digestion process.

Some people naturally have a higher or lower enzyme activity. Aside from enzymes, an even more natural way to improve digestion is to incorporate a digestive aid in the morning and evening, such as warm lemon water with a splash of apple cider vinegar. This can be a beginning and end of the day ritual that primes your digestion and facilitates the elimination of toxins.

DEGLYCERIZED LICORICE (DGL) has been known to soothe the mucosal gut lining and balance stomach acid secretion. Licorice root is truly of the kind as it has many uses, including for hormonal, gut, and respiratory issues. The deglycerized licorice version has the majority of the glycyrrhizin component removed to prevent a common side effect, which is hypertension. Aside from being able to soothe the gut, DGL also helps with common complaints like heartburn, gastritis, and peptic ulcer disease.[29]

There are many other supplements to talk about, but these are enough for starters. I mentioned that food comes first and supplements second. I'd like to end this section by providing a comprehensive food elimination outline as well as a step by step guide for reintroducing foods at the end of the challenge. Having an optimally functioning digestive system can help with cravings by creating a healthy environment for gut bacteria to thrive in. As with everything else, quality matters. Be sure that your supplements and food are of the highest quality. Choose organic and non-genetically modified as often as you can. Your health is worth it.

►CHAPTER 5 EXERCISES: Food Elimination & Reintroduction of Gluten, Dairy, Corn, Soy Egg, Citrus Fruits, Sugar, Food Additives, and Alcohol

Before considering starting an elimination challenge, answer the following questions below to see if this is something you can benefit from:

1. Do you experience gas/bloating on a regular basis?
2. Do you feel that you often skip a bowel movement and are not regular?
3. Do you experience frequent digestive upset?

4. Have you had frequent antibiotic use?
5. At any point in time, did you consume a high amount of sugar and/or artificial sweeteners?
6. Do you have frequent yeast infections, urinary tract infections, or skin breakouts, or do you experience pain and inflammation on a regular basis?

If you answered YES to any of these, working on improving gut health can be highly beneficial.

The purpose of the elimination diet is to clear the body of foods that may be causing or aggravating your symptoms, including food cravings. This process will help identify any hidden food sensitivities or allergies and improve your health and well-being. There are three main steps to a successful elimination diet.

Step 1: PLAN

It's best to do this challenge for minimum of six weeks in order to give your immune system a chance to reset. You may choose to work with your healthcare provider to learn which foods might be causing problems. It also may be useful to keep a food journal prior to beginning your elimination to keep track of the foods you are currently eating and your symptoms throughout the day. Often it is the foods that you crave or those you consume most frequently that are considered for elimination challenge.

Before moving on to the elimination phase, create a clear plan detailing the foods that you will avoid. Determine your "allowed foods" and gather recipes and resources to ensure success during your elimination.

Step 2: ELIMINATE

Follow the elimination diet without exceptions for at least **SIX WEEKS** and consume only allowed foods during this time.

Read Labels: Examine all labels carefully to look for hidden ingredients.

For example, if you are avoiding dairy products, you need to check labels for **whey, casein, and lactose**. Be particularly cautious if you are eating out, since you have less control of what goes into your food. **When in doubt, ASK!** Restaurants are very aware and accommodating these days.

Food Quality: You may get better results with the elimination diet if you drink purified water and eat only organic, pesticide free produce, legumes, and grains. Choose organic, pastured, or grass fed meats. Avoid artificial ingredients, added colors, hydrogenated oils, and deep-fried foods.

Troubling Symptoms: Withdrawal symptoms may occur during the first few days or weeks on the diet. Some or all of your symptoms may increase temporarily. It is also possible to experience new symptoms. These symptoms may be lessened by:

- Drinking at least eight glasses of purified water a day.
- Taking baths with Epsom salts.
- Napping for no more than fifteen to twenty minutes to keep your circadian rhythm balanced.
- Exercise—Movement is great way to take your mind off things, refresh your body, and support good digestion as well as detoxification.

SOME TIPS:

A food elimination challenge normally has a low compliance rate, because the list of foods to be eliminated is long. Start an elimination challenge by eliminating several foods at a time. Begin by eliminating foods like dairy, gluten, and products containing processed sugar for a few weeks, reintroduce them, watch for any negative mental, emotional, or physical symptoms, and repeat with other foods on the elimination list.

You will find two things surprising during the elimination challenge: 1) how hard it is to give something up (this goes back to Chapter 1 and understanding the addictive nature of food) and 2) how great you feel giving up certain foods like sugar.

	FOOD TO INCLUDE	FOOD TO EXCLUDE
Grains	Non-gluten grains: rice (preferably whole grain), quinoa, buckwheat, millet, amaranth, teff	Corn, wheat, barley, rye, oats **(except "gluten-free" oats)**, bulgur, couscous, pasta (except "gluten free"), durum, einkorn, emmer, faro, graham, kamut, semolina, spelt, triticale
Fruit	Pears and apples	Citrus: oranges, grapefruits, lemons, and limes
Protein	Lamb, chicken, pork, grass fed beef, fish, wild game meats, such as venison, all beans and legumes except peanuts and soybeans	Shellfish, processed meats, such as cold cuts, canned meats, hot dogs and sausage, eggs, dairy products, all soy products including tempeh, tofu, edamame, soy milk
Dairy	Rice milk, nut and seed milks, such as almond, hazelnut, hemp, amazake, coconut milk,	All animal milks (goat, sheep, cow), all cheeses, butter, ghee, cream, kefir, yogurt, casein, whey, soy yogurt, soy cheese
Vegetables	All raw, steamed, sautéed, juiced or roasted/baked vegetables	Corn, creamed vegetables, nightshade vegetables (tomatoes, potatoes, bell peppers, cayenne, eggplant)
Nuts and seeds	All nuts and seeds are allowed, except peanuts (which is a legume and not a nut)	
Oils/Fats	All oils except butter, corn, and soybean oil. Preferred oils include: Cold pressed extra virgin olive oil, flax seed oil, walnut oil, sesame oil, coconut oil	Corn and soybean oils, butter, ghee

Sweeteners	Maple syrup, honey, stevia, **in small amounts**	White/brown sugars, corn syrup, barley malt, high fructose corn syrup, evaporated cane juice/sucanat, all artificial sweeteners
Beverages	Water (plain, mineral, or sparkling), herbal teas, fresh squeezed juice with added pulp	hot chocolate, dairy, alcoholic beverages, soda, and decrease caffeine intake
Condiments	Salt, black pepper, herbs, spices, vinegar, garlic, onions, coconut aminos	Chocolate, soy sauce, mayonnaise, ketchup made with corn syrup, teriyaki sauce

Reintroduction of Foods—Identifying the Culprits

The purpose of reintroducing foods or challenging them after six weeks is to help you determine which foods might be causing negative symptoms. The reintroduction challenge consists of a one-day challenge in which you will reintroduce an eliminated food to your diet, followed by a one-day symptom observation. This two-day process is repeated for each food you reintroduce to your diet.

Directions:

Eat two to three average size servings of a pure form of your challenge food through the course of one day. A pure form is a food that does not have additives or other ingredients that you have been omitting from your diet (e.g. sugar or artificial colorants).

Pure food examples:
- A piece of whole wheat toast (plain)
- A glass of whole milk
- Egg yolk and egg white (try one then the other)
- A whole tomato

- Corn on the cob (plain)
- Tofu (plain)

After your one-day challenge, take the challenged food back out of your diet. Regardless of your reaction, you will keep this food out of your diet until the end of the reintroduction phase. Observe your reactions for two days. This gives you time to notice both immediate and delayed reactions. Record food intake and observations. Write down anything that feels different from when you were in the full elimination phase of the diet. Potential reactions may include: **skin irritations or breakout, gas, bloating, abdominal pain, diarrhea or constipation, headache, fatigue, depression, anxiety, muscle or join pain.** Repeat the above directions for each food group.

Chapter 6
The Chemical Messengers: Our Hormones

"What we now know is there are very real hormonal factors involved. It's not just your genetics, willpower, or eating habits. What it takes to balance the weight equation that leaves so many women struggling, is a balancing act of each of these elements."

—DR. MARCELLE PICK, FOUNDER OF WOMEN TO WOMEN: TRANSFORMING WOMEN'S HEALTH NATURALLY

If you've ever been to an orchestra concert, you've seen how the large instrumental ensemble of violin, cello, brass, woodwinds, and other instruments are grouped in sections and led by the conductor. The conductor directs the performance, sets the tempo of the music, and provides instructions to the musicians with the intention of delivering music that's unified and pleasant to listen to.

Your body is similar to an orchestra. The cells that make up the body are the musicians with their different roles and functions. Hormones, the messengers that are secreted into the blood stream by various glands, such as the thyroid or adrenal gland, are the conductors that tell the cells what to do. In a healthy individual, the cells receive the messages from the hormones and act accordingly. But when there is a hormonal imbalance and the cells no longer respond to the messages, or they are not receiving the messages due to a hormone deficiency, or they don't know what to do with the messages, the music in our body becomes chaotic and no longer as unified as that of a perfectly orchestrated system.

Hormones have different roles and functions, and their deficiency or abundance can cause symptoms similar to and different from nutrient deficiencies. I won't cover all the hormones and what they do here but will discuss the role of thyroid and adrenal glands that can directly influence our cravings, which can help us identify if they are off balance.

One of my patients came to see me because she was struggling to lose weight no matter what she did. She was at the point of frustration—cutting calories didn't work, and exercising over five times a week was not working either. In my practice, I never just target weight loss, as that is almost secondary. Sure, there are cases where that is the sole primary objective, but rarely is that the only issue. This patient also complained about unusual hair loss, loss of energy, and severe sugar cravings, which she minimized at first because she was so focused on the weight loss component.

Then there was the question of libido or sexual drive. "What libido?" she would jokingly say. My patient was so focused on weight loss that all the other symptoms were like background noise—bothersome, yet tolerable, although eventually they would become unbearable. Of course, I wanted to help her lose weight, but my primary objective was to get her feeling better and identify the root cause of the symptoms paired with unwanted weight gain. Everything else would follow.

The two key hormone-producing glands that often contribute to unwanted weight gain, hair loss, and food cravings are the thyroid and adrenal glands. I often refer to the thyroid gland as our furnace, as it is responsible for how well or poorly our metabolism functions. When people think of metabolism, they frequently associate it with weight loss or weight gain—which is just part of the equation. Metabolism, however, is more than just how quickly you metabolize food. It involves all the biochemical processes in the body—everything from digestion and absorption to waste removal and optimal cellular function. The thyroid hormones T4 and T3 are the big players with a big impact on our metabolism, but frequently their deficiency gets overlooked.

The big problem in the medical community is that patients and providers rely on just the lab tests to help identify a thyroid problem. Patients are not the ones to blame, as they rely on the guidance of physicians. I've seen numerous cases where patients come in with lab results that their provider did not explain, or their provider said the results are "normal" and there's nothing more to look at. Even if the results are "normal," if you are experiencing any of the classical symptoms of decreased metabolism, such as constipation, cold intolerance, weight gain, mental fog, sleepiness, dry skin, or hair loss, your thyroid may not be functioning optimally.

Early symptoms of thyroid problems can seem like the symptoms of everyday life, and many cases of thyroid disease go undiagnosed or are mistaken for other conditions. One of the biggest complaints people have, along with the other symptoms, is the craving for sugar. Low thyroid function decreases the rate of glucose uptake by cells and the rate of glucose absorption in the gut, slows the insulin response to glucose in the bloodstream, such as after a meal, and also slows the clearance of insulin from the bloodstream after it has done its job. All of these are signs of a slowed metabolism that can have you going after sugar like a cupcake monster.

The common symptoms of hypoglycemia or low blood sugar include fatigue, headache, hunger, and irritability. When your cells are not getting the sugar they need, this puts pressure on the adrenal glands. The adrenals release the stress hormone called cortisol in order to increase the amount of glucose available to the cells. So unless we improve thyroid function, your body will be in a vicious cycle of being hypoglycemic, secreting cortisol, and contributing to higher stress levels that in turn further suppress the thyroid function—a no longer perfectly orchestrated system.

So, although your lab results may show normal levels of glucose in the bloodstream, you'll still have symptoms of hypoglycemia— fatigue, headache, hunger, shakiness, and irritability. And since your cells aren't getting the glucose they need, your adrenals will release cortisol to increase the amount of glucose available to them. This causes the chronic stress response described above, which further stresses the thyroid.

The big question is why does this big mess happen?

The psychological and physical demands of daily life, such as school, work, sleepless nights, emotional stress, and dieting, put significant demand on our adrenal glands, which in turn produce cortisol to help us stay awake, alert, and ready for the next challenge of the day. Think of it this way: If you are driving down the highway at 60 mph, eventually you'll start running out of gas, and no matter how hard you press on the gas pedal, the car won't go any farther and will come to a screeching halt. Classic cases of an adrenal imbalance are observed in athletes who overtrain, students who stay up late and get up early, sleep-deprived parents, and busy professionals clocking in and clocking out without ever seeing the sun. Does this sound familiar?

Like a car's gas tank, which gets depleted after a certain amount of time, the adrenal glands become impaired in their ability to help us manage the daily stressors of life, especially when everything around us is moving at a rapid pace. As adrenal function declines, it fails to produce the other essential hormones to our well-being, such as DHEA and the sex hormones estrogen, progesterone, and testosterone. At this point, uncontrollable cravings for both sugar and salt become significant, among other symptoms, such as low libido, weight gain around the thighs and abdomen, and fatigue, to name just a few.[32]

My patient who was desperate to lose weight was not even considering a possible hormone imbalance as a cause for how she was feeling. For all she knew, it all had to do with her diet and exercise, as her labs kept coming back "normal." I see this happen all the time in both women and men. Unfortunately, because providers in the conventional medical system are preoccupied with catching something that is obviously wrong (there's a time and place for this, too), they frequently overlook signs and symptoms of a potential disorder or imbalance that can be easily treated. So, unless your labs are below or above normal, you're considered to be fine, and it's part of getting older. Let's bust this myth, because it is so not true!

Although adrenal fatigue is not recognized as an official disease in the medical community, the conglomerate of symptoms that appear in patients should not be dismissed and taken lightly. Both the adrenal and thyroid gland play a vital role in our well-being. When these two glands start to malfunction from being overworked, we start to see an array of physical, mental, and emotional symptoms, including severe food cravings that don't go away. The good news is that there are many natural treatments that can help restore the normal function of these two important hormone glands, help reset cravings, and get you back on the path to optimal health.

Effective treatments should aim to address all aspects of mental, emotional, and physical health. Although the following recommendations can help with symptoms of thyroid and adrenal imbalance, it is always important to consult with your physician before starting any treatment and to rule out any other contributing or serious conditions.

The diet is always one of the most important areas to start with. When it comes to adrenal and thyroid health, a diet rich in healthy fats is of utmost importance. Healthy fats – such as coconut oil, avocados, nuts and seeds, and fatty fish – are nutrient superfoods and can help restore the nervous system by balancing blood sugar, supporting brain function, and providing the essential nutrients for proper hormone synthesis.[33] Another important aspect of the diet is the timing between meals. Having more frequent, smaller meals – four to six a day – is a much better and more efficient way to fuel your tank rather than having three large meals. Your blood sugar will be balanced throughout the day, and you'll be less likely to binge on something when the vending machine is calling your name.

Caffeine is also something to address. People suffering from fatigue due to adrenal or thyroid causes frequently reach for coffee to fight off excess fatigue. One of the biggest mistakes people make is skipping breakfast and having coffee on an empty stomach. Physiologically, caffeine has a sympathetic response on the nervous system. It causes an increase in heart rate and blood pressure and releases cortisol. Small amounts of caffeine have health-boosting properties, but in a person suffering from adrenal fatigue, caffeine can make the situation worse. Caffeine makes the overworked adrenals produce more cortisol when the gland is already deprived, stressing it even further.

The *Adrenal Fatigue Solution*, written by Fawne Hansen and fellow naturopath Dr. Eric Wood, has a clear explanation of the impact that caffeine has on the nervous system and hormones. Caffeine stimulates the brain to alert the adrenal glands that they need to pump out more adrenaline and cortisol. This puts you in a fight or flight mode, a sympathetic nervous system response that gets triggered every time you drink a cup of coffee. One cup may not necessarily cause so much distress, and coffee does have benefits, but most people run into trouble when one cup turns into three.

I experienced this after my son was born. I woke up four to six times per night for the first six months, juggled a busy private practice, and was running a business. There was not enough time in the day to do my job, and the coffee would lure me in after the 4 a.m. wake up call each morning. I hired the most amazing sleep consultant, Marianne Jacobson, to help me figure out my son's sleep schedule, and she pointed out something that hadn't occurred to me. My son was running on the same adrenaline and cortisol that I was. My lifestyle, and coffee that came with it, wasn't helping his sleep or mine. As you can imagine, I personally had to reinvent my schedule and decrease my dependency on coffee.

The adrenal gland serves a primitive purpose. Its essential role is to avoid harm or danger through the fight or flight mechanism of cortisol production and to support reproduction by pumping out sex hormones. I often joke that in the caveman era, you would want to run away from the saber-toothed tiger (cortisol) before you could reproduce (sex hormones). Another important piece to this is that the adrenal gland will always use its building blocks to produce cortisol first before it will produce sex hormones. What I frequently find in comprehensive hormone tests is that usually the sex hormones start to decline, but cortisol levels remain almost normal. That's because all attention is allocated to producing this stress hormone—a piece of the puzzle that gets overlooked frequently in the context of both patient symptoms and lab results.

My superstar patient, who was conquering the gym religiously and throwing every possible diet at her body, found out that she, in fact, had a lower than normal thyroid function together with elevated cortisol and a decrease in the major sex hormones. Within weeks of treatment for both thyroid and adrenal imbalances, she had more energy and fewer sugar cravings, and she was on her way to losing weight. To my delight, she actually started to care more about how great she felt than how much she weighed—a truly refreshing and much welcomed approach to health!

I can't talk about hormones without talking about lifestyle. Given the role that cortisol plays, in trying to restore both thyroid and adrenal function, it's important to understand the stress management component. We move through life at a rapid rate without taking the time to take care of our overworked minds and bodies. The amount of research done regarding stress and its negative effects as well as the benefits of stress management is tremendous. Stress reduction has been proven to improve general well-being, increase performance, boost immunity, and help in managing cravings as well as weight loss.[35]

When you find yourself craving comfort food because you are overworked, stressed out, or had little sleep, choose an activity that can help you destress and energize naturally – such as a brisk walk or a short meditation session – before reaching for the bag of chips or cookies. It can also be helpful to plan smaller meals throughout the day as mentioned earlier. Include meals rich in lean protein, healthy fats, vegetables, and fruit to keep energy levels optimal, keep blood sugar stable, and decrease the likelihood of the afternoon crash.

In my personal and professional life, I try to guide clients, friends, and family to make the best snack and meal decisions. Snacks during the day are often where people struggle, so planning becomes essential. I fill my social media with pictures of my go-to snacks, and I've received a lot of feedback from friends and clients alike, telling me that it helps them make their decisions. A lot of times, my snacks are planned, but frequently, I am just like everyone else wandering into a store trying to find something healthy and nutritious to snack on amid work and errands. I think of myself as a professional snacker, because it's taken me years to know what works, what doesn't, what are the best food combinations, and what to reach for when in a hurry.

Aside from diet and stress management, there are specific nutrients available in supplement form that can help thyroid and adrenal glands work more efficiently. The key nutrients for the thyroid include selenium, iodine, and botanicals, such as kelp or seaweed, Ashwagandha, Blue Flag root, Myrr Gum, Nettles, Triphala, and Ginger. For adrenal health, nutrients, such as B Vitamins, particularly B-6, B-5, and B12, Magnesium, L-Carnitine, and Vitamin C, are important. You will also find that adrenal-supporting formulas will contain herbal preparations consisting of botanicals, such as holy basil leaf, hawthorne leaf and flower, eleuthero root, alfalfa herb, and rhodiola root. All of these are meant to provide basic support for the glands and should always be taken as prescribed by your healthcare provider.

Although many thyroid and adrenal support formulas are available over the counter and can be purchased in many different stores, including online, I'd like to say a word of caution. It is always wise to consult your physician first, especially if you are having any possible symptoms of a thyroid or adrenal problem.

Many conditions have similar symptoms. Taking herbal and nutrient preparations without first identifying the problem or ruling out the potential risks of taking supplements can be dangerous. Since many people are also usually on some sort of a pharmaceutical agent that can interfere with supplements and vice versa, it is best to consult with your provider to ensure product safety. The supplement industry has become saturated with many players, many of whom slap labels onto products that have little research and quality assurance. The internet has made it easy to connect buyers and sellers, and, as a doctor and someone who does prescribe supplements, I like to educate everyone about the importance of knowing the source and quality of what you're taking.

The end of this chapter provides you with a list of questions to think about regarding thyroid and adrenal gland health. Avoid diagnosing yourself—these questions are meant to be more of a guide. Because diet is such an important and fundamental building block to longevity, after the questions, I've provided recipes that help support your thyroid and adrenals on a daily basis. Prevention is the best medicine!

Note that if you are someone who is suffering from adrenal fatigue, it can take months and years to recover completely. That is how significant this is. When talking to my clients, I always bring up the Yerkes–Dodson curve, which shows the relationship between arousal and performance and was originally developed by psychologists Robert M. Yerkes and John Dillingham Dodson in 1908. The curve shows that initially performance increases with physiological or mental arousal, but only up to a point—the point of diminishing returns. Past this point, additional arousal or stress creates a decrease in performance. No matter how much you input, your output starts to decrease. The issue with adrenal fatigue is that even when the stressor is gone, once someone is past the point of diminishing returns, it can be really hard to bounce back and start feeling normal. As with all good things in life, it takes time, patience, and a lot of good self-care.

►**CHAPTER 6 EXERCISES:** The Basic Hormone Test &
Recipes for Optimal Hormone Health

1. Questions relating to Adrenal Function:

- Do you feel exhausted and stressed most of the time?
- Do you need a constant caffeine boost to make it through the day?
- Do you have trouble waking up, falling asleep, or staying asleep, or wake up not feeling refreshed?
- Do you find yourself feeling constantly irritable?
- Do you feel exhausted after working out?
- Do you feel as though everything you eat turns to fat?
- Are you always hungry or frequently craving carbohydrates, salt, and sugar?
- Are you plagued by irregular or painful periods or PMS?
- Are you struggling with a low libido?
- Do you find yourself feeling forgetful or "foggy" or unable to concentrate?

Answering yes to any of these questions can indicate an adrenal dysfunction.

Follow the guidelines above to help improve symptoms and regain your life.

2. Questions relating to Thyroid Function:

- Do you have difficulty losing weight?
- Do you have cold hands and feet or are you sensitive to cold?
- Do you have difficulty thinking or concentrating?
- Do you have poor short-term memory?
- Are your moods depressed?
- Are you experiencing hair loss, eye brow thinning, or brittle hair and nails?

- Do you have fewer that one BM per day?
- Do you have dry skin?
- Do you have fluid retention?
- Do you have recurrent headaches?
- Are you tired when you awaken?
- Have you had infertility or miscarriages (2)?
- Do you have muscle aches or joint pain?
- Have you had recurrent infections?

As you can see, there are overlaps between the thyroid and adrenal gland questions. Answering yes to any of the above questions can point to a thyroid and/or adrenal dysfunction. Often, treating both the thyroid and adrenals is essential to correcting the imbalance and symptoms.

Everyday Recipes for Optimal Hormone Health:

You guys are in for a treat! When it comes to adrenal and thyroid health, optimal fuel is key. If you suffer or have ever suffered with adrenal fatigue or have had issues with your thyroid, you know that maintaining well-balanced sugar is challenging yet important.

Having experience with overtraining, going through medical school, opening my own business, and giving birth to our first baby, all within a few years, I would find myself crashing, reaching for foods that I normally wouldn't (oh, the cravings!), and eating lunch at 10 a.m. Have you ever experienced that?

The more nutrient dense your meals are, the better you will feel, recover, and see results in your personal health. I can't stress enough how planning for these meals is a HUGE component to all of this and is a lifestyle makeover that pays off big-time in the long run.

You'll notice a few key ingredients in these recipes and may wonder **why in the heck are things like avocado, coconut oil, and maca in almost every recipe?** I found that these ingredients are the most nutrient-dense foods that give the best results. You don't have to have avocado with every meal, obviously, so feel free to substitute it with nuts or anything else that you prefer.

The key here is healthy fats and a balance between protein and carbohydrates. Thyroid and adrenal issues are best mitigated with a balance of fat, protein, and carbohydrates. Too much or too little of any of these macronutrients and your body will give you symptoms in the form of cravings, digestion issues, fatigue, low energy, changes in appetite, etc. It's a fine dance, and you're the choreographer!

Play with these and other recipes in this book, and fine tune them to meet your taste palette. For me personally, I have used the smoothies and scones for breakfast, as a snack, and as a treat before bed. (You do sleep better when you have a snack before bed, another fun piece of information.) You may choose not to have the whole serving. For example, if after dinner I want dessert, I'll make a smoothie a little thicker and put it in a bowl and eat it with a spoon. If a few hours have gone by since dinner and I need a quick snack after working and tucking my baby to sleep, then I'll have a couple of bites of a buckwheat scone with a tablespoon of nut butter. I also like the scones first thing in the morning when I wake up hungry but need to squeeze in a workout. I will grab a couple of bites to get my blood sugar back up and give me the energy to start and finish my workout.

I hope these examples will help you make the best choices during the day and provide you with some insight on how to use these recipes.

*

Power Smoothie, Anytime:

Makes 1 smoothie

1 scoop vanilla protein powder

2 tsp spirulina

1/2 frozen banana

1/2 avocado

1/2 cup of frozen blueberries

1 Tbsp of coconut cream

1/4 Tbsp Himalayan pink salt

1 cup of coconut or other nut milk

Place all ingredients in a blender and blend until smooth. Add more liquid as necessary. Enjoy first thing in the morning or any time of the day when you're craving something sweet.

Vibrant Gluten Free Oats

Makes 2 servings

1 cup gluten free oats

2 cups coconut milk

2 tsp Maca Powder

1 scoop of vanilla protein

1 Tbsp coconut oil

1 Tbsp maple syrup

pinch of Himalayan salt

Bring coconut milk to a boil and add the oats. Turn heat to low and let cook for 5 minutes or until oats are done, depending on the brand. Turn the heat off and add the maca powder, protein, coconut oil, and maple syrup. Add salt to taste.

Green Goddess Salad

Makes 4-6 servings

6 cups of spinach

1 green apple, chopped

1/4 cup of sunflower seeds

1/2 cup of walnuts

1/4 cup of hemp seeds

2 Tbsp Honey

1/4 tsp Black pepper

1/2 tsp of Himalayan Salt

4 Tbsp Apple cider vinegar

1/4 cup Avocado or Olive Oil

Prewash spinach and dry using a spinner, paper towels, or a towel. Toss in the apple, walnuts, sunflower seeds, and hemp seeds. Combine the oil with the vinegar, salt, pepper, and honey by whisking briskly or using a blender. Pour the dressing over the salad and serve! You can pair this salad with a protein of your choice, such as chicken, salmon, tofu, or anything else that strikes you! It goes well with hearty grains like quinoa as well. If you want to make ahead and don't want the spinach to be soggy, substitute kale, which will soak up the dressing and will actually be better the next day, as its texture is tougher.

Fuel Buckwheat Scones

1 Tbsp ground flaxseed meal (egg alternative!)

2 1/2 Tbsp water

1/4 cup raw honey or maple syrup

1/4 cup coconut oil, melted

4 Tbsp of nut milk, such as coconut milk

1 3/4 cup buckwheat flour

1 tsp gluten-free baking powder

2 tsp lemon zest

1 tsp chopped fresh rosemary, optional

Pinch of salt

Pre-heat oven to 350°F and line a baking sheet with parchment paper. Combine flaxseed meal with water to create a flax egg. In a large mixing bowl, mix honey and coconut oil together, and then add flax egg and nut milk of choice and mix until combined. In a separate bowl, combine buckwheat flour, baking powder, lemon zest, and chopped rosemary. Add dry ingredients to the bowl with the wet ingredients and mix until you get a thick, even consistency cookie dough. Shape the dough into a circle and place on the prepared baking sheet. Slice the dough into 6 pieces (scone shape) and separate each piece leaving 2 inches of space between each piece. Bake scones for 10 to 12 minutes, until scones are golden brown on the bottom. Baking time will vary depending on your oven. (I tried this recipe in a different oven and it took 20 minutes.) Serve scones warm with coconut oil or ghee.

Sea Monster Salad
Makes 4 servings

Salad:

1 large head or 4 cups of curly kale, stems removed and leaves chopped

1/2 avocado, pitted and cubed

1 medium sized cucumber, cubed

4 Tbsp wakame seaweed

2 Tbsp of sesame seeds

Dressing:

1-1/2 avocados, pitted with skins removed

2 garlic cloves

Juice from 1 lemon

1/4 cup cilantro

3 Tbsp sesame seed oil

1 tsp Apple Cider vinegar

1/2 tsp ground chipotle pepper

Himalayan Salt to taste

Cover the dried seaweed with water and let sit for 5 minutes until it softens. Rinse with cool water. Place all dressing ingredients in a blender and process until smooth. Adjust seasoning and liquids as necessary. Place the chopped kale pieces in a bowl, pour a few tablespoons of the dressing over the leaves, and massage with your hands until the fibers in the leaves begin to break down and it starts to soften. Add the cucumber, avocado, and seaweed to the salad, and add more dressing to taste. Sprinkle with sesame seeds. You may have some of the dressing leftover, but you can save it to add to salad the next day or to another salad another time!

Chapter 7:
The Environmental Influence

"Whenever you find yourself on the side of the majority, it is time to pause and reflect."

— MARK TWAIN

A host of internal factors impact our everyday decisions around food—brain chemistry, genetics, wacky hormones, and hungry gut bacteria. But aside from our inner landscape, the outside environment serves a distinct role in shaping our desires and triggers for food. In this chapter, we dive into some of the common influences, including work, social, and family environments.

A lot of my clients struggle with in-office meeting lunches, team parties and events, and break-room snacking and feel judged for the food decisions they make, particularly when they are good ones. Clients have reported that they found it difficult to refuse a cookie offered by a co-worker, experienced a sense of discomfort saying no to pasta at social events, and felt insecure about their healthy choices when everyone around them was ordering junk food. "What will people think, or what should I do if they ask me why I eat the way I do?" are common questions, and I do a lot of counseling to get past that.

In social psychology, the term "herd mentality" describes how people choose to adopt certain behaviors based on the influence of their peers. We can observe herd mentality in stock market trends, housing bubbles, consumer behavior, and sporting events. This phenomenon is not new to humankind. Historically, herd mentality along with herd behavior was a survival mechanism by which tribes formed, migrated, and performed group tasks that had a cooperative impact.[36] Because herd mentality plays such an important role in our day-to-day decisions, its impact on the choices we make around food is undeniable.

There is plenty of research done around the herd mentality phenomenon and the way it impacts our behavior. For instance, the results of an experiment done by researchers from the Leeds University showed that it only takes about 5% of confident-looking and instructed people to influence the direction of the other 95%. Professor Krause and a PhD student John Dyer conducted a series of experiments where groups of people were asked to walk randomly around a large hall. A select few within the group received more detailed instructions about where to walk. Participants were not allowed to communicate with one another but had to stay within arm's length of another person. The findings show that in all cases, the informed individuals were followed by others in the crowd, forming self-organizing units. What's interesting is that Professor Krause noticed that most individuals didn't even realize that they were doing this.[37]

I am sure most of us can recall an example of herd mentality from our own lives. Take, for example, going out to a restaurant. One person will start to order a burger and fries, someone else orders a cobb salad loaded with bacon and blue cheese with a soda or a beer, and then there are appetizers for the whole table. In my private practice, I have had patients tell me that they feel awkward when they go out to a restaurant with a group of friends and have to modify items on the menu to meet their dietary needs. Instead, they resort to ordering "safe" foods to avoid being judged or have to explain themselves to the group. "I just hate being that person," many of my clients say.

In my personal health, I have struggled with the herd mentality around food as well. I've been questioned, made fun of, and even critiqued by acquaintances and friends, because after being sugar and crave free for over a decade, I rarely compromise. I believe in long-term results that require long-term commitment, so for me to "slip," there's a lot that needs to go wrong. It takes months and sometimes years to develop your own system that works for you. I know how I feel when I don't have junk food and how I feel when I do. My life is built around performance and helping others achieve peak health, so every meal and every decision I make during the day either brings me closer to feeling great or does the opposite.

When going out, I try not to deviate too much from my normal diet, and I frequently find myself being that person who orders the burger without the bun (honestly, I couldn't care less for it!), or limiting cheese and dressings on my salads, or saying "no, thank you" to a co-worker's home baked cookies—sorry—I work too hard to say yes to that, and frankly, I've gone so long without eating processed foods that it doesn't even taste the same. However, if it's home baked cookies with honey instead of sugar and almond or coconut flour instead of white or wheat flour, and if the cookie is filled with healthy fats like nuts and hemp protein....then you have my attention!

For the past five years, my mother-in-law kept buying cake and bringing treats to our house, insisting that we have some. It took that long to convince her to stop trying to get me to eat cake. I don't eat it. Period. I used to feel bad about saying no, but what I have learned is that saying no has become easier then saying yes. Brené Brown, the leading researcher in the concepts of vulnerability, courage, empathy, and shame, talks about the impact of saying yes instead of no in *The Power of Vulnerability*. We say yes because saying no feels uncomfortable in the moment. We say yes, even though we know it's not really how we feel. Saying yes to something that does not resonate with us in the moment has consequences: guilt, dissatisfaction, and then frustration. I can't thank Brené enough for the impact her work has had in shaping my day-to-day experiences.

Back to the cake. The problem is not in the cake per se but in the ingredients that are often used. This is the point that I am trying to drive. Have your cake, your cookies, your ice cream, but pay attention to the ingredients that go in there. A cookie made from the wholesome ingredients I mentioned earlier is not going to contribute to diabetes or irregular blood sugar or freak out your digestion. It will work for your health rather than against it.

What about those once or twice a year (maybe even more frequently) occasions like holidays or birthdays?

One of my clients knows that when she eats processed sugar, she gets irritable and anxious, and it fuels her cravings for sugar. For her, even a bite is not worth being in this state. However, there is one day in the year when her mom comes to visit, and they make these special sugar cookies. To say she loves the whole process of making them is an understatement. The experience she shares with her mom, the smell of the baked cookies, and the taste take her back to her childhood. This is really the only time during the year when she wants to give in, and she should! Because the problem is not in saying yes to a treat on special occasions or once in a while but in how frequently we say yes and at what cost to our health.

Our decisions around food are largely shaped by the social environment we find ourselves in. Motivational speaker Jim Rohn is known for saying that we are the average of the five people we spend the most time with. We are affected by our environment more than we think, and our decisions are greatly influenced by the people closest to us. Maybe now is a good time to pause and reflect. Who are the people in your life who shape some of your behaviors around food, exercise, and general lifestyle choices?

An excellent example of a community coming together to take charge of their health and support one another in making better decisions around nutrition and lifestyle is in the Daniel Plan, founded by the best-selling author of the *Purpose Driven Life* and Pastor to Saddleback Church, Rick Warren, and a group of leading medical experts, Dr. Mark Hyman, Dr. Mehmet Oz, and Dr. Daniel Amen. The Daniel Plan was created to help church members live a healthier life at the time when Pastor Rick Warren was noticing that too many of the church's members were overweight. The plan included individual, group, and weekend service participation to help people get the support and empowerment they needed. With this level of accountability on an individual and group level, the church was able to lose thousands of pounds, as Dr. Hyman would later recall during an interview.

The Daniel Plan called this community experience of living a healthy life the "Power of Alignment." Individuals congregated to support one another in the spirit of a better life, a life that combined faith, nutrition, community, fitness, and the right psychology to help people succeed.[38] That sounds like a winning formula.

In addition to day-to-day social interactions that can impact cravings and decisions around food, other environmental factors influence what we crave and how much we eat. These other factors, such as packaging, lighting, situational cues, and the surrounding environment, can influence our consumption volume by suggesting an alternative consumption normal. The holiday season is a great example of how the country as a whole can deviate from normal consumption.

Consider the end-of-year weight gain that many experience between Thanksgiving, Christmas, and New Year's holidays. This weight gain can be attributed to both the eating environment (i.e. eating with others and eating distractions) and the food environment (i.e. salience of food, size of food packages and portions). The holiday eating environment encourages overconsumption because it involves parties with long eating durations, holiday parties spaced close together, family gatherings with all sorts of food varieties, plenty of leftovers, eating with others, and a multitude of distractions. So before you know it, instead of having one plate, you're having three, and this cycle repeats itself through the holiday season. It's kind of like eating at a buffet for three months. To top it off, research has shown that the prominence and stockpiles of food typically found at holiday parties further fuel overconsumption.[40]

Because I'm on a mission to help you experience the joy of good health in a way that is sustainable and replicable in any environment, I've provided hearty, delicious, and holiday-friendly recipes that everyone can enjoy. You can feel good about these recipes and cook them for potlucks, parties, and events. Moreover, in case of leftovers, they are not loaded with sugar, salt, and processed fats that you're eating for days. Most of my patients are always asking about meal ideas and recipe suggestions, so I thought I'd include some of my favorite go-to's.

Aside from the holiday environment, what about the office work space? Most break rooms are filled with sugary and salty foods like chips, crackers, cookies, and donuts that someone brings to a meeting. I've done enough workspace audits to know that's the case in most situations, even in the most progressive of companies. Even in my own office space, someone usually sneaks in cookies, a colleague will bring a box of donuts, or we have tons of post-party snacks that lay around waiting for a hungry victim to come by—myself included!

Combine holiday celebrations with someone's birthday at the office, and you have a perfect storm of candy flooding the countertops and birthday cake creating a wave-like sugar crash from one person to the next. The typical workspace can be a deadly combination of sitting in one place for hours and overconsuming processed, salty, and sugary snacks to cure boring meetings and manage stress. Not to mention the peer pressure to partake in the donuts, which are endlessly floating around office meeting tables. Temptation is on every corner, as many of my patients describe their work environment. The good news is that you can beat the office sugar blues and ignore the sirens from the vending machine by following some of the following tips:

BRING YOUR GO-TO SNACKS TO THE OFFICE

A lot of people are caught off-guard when they come into the break room or get done with a lengthy meeting. Failing to plan ahead is the number one mistake when it comes to nutrition. So, plan to succeed by prepping your snacks the night before. Even if you have an impromptu meeting, a colleague distracts you from your lunch, or you don't even get a lunch—if you have something handy in your bag, desk, or workplace refrigerator, your taste buds and your waistline will thank you. Refer to the recipes at the end of this chapter for ideas on food that you can bring to the office—for yourself and others! After all, sharing is caring, especially when it's good food.

PRACTICE SAYING "NO, THANK YOU"

This will probably be the hardest part. We are raised to clear our plates and say yes when anyone offers us anything, and we feel guilty knowing that people in other parts of the world don't have the luxury to say no—all very real and very valid thoughts. The issue here is not about saying yes but about the overabundance of saying yes to people and food that, in the end, makes us sick. Food is personal, and the moment you start saying "no, thank you" to the birthday cake, to the baked cookies, or to the donuts being passed around the meeting table, people will start to question your judgement. It has happened to me many times and to my clients as well. You know the chemical cascade of reactions that sugary and processed snacks create, but the offering party may not. Simply saying something along the lines of, "I am actually really content right now" or even simpler, "No, thank you" without explanation will work.

BRING JUNK FOOD ALTERNATIVES TO WORK MEETINGS:

Set a New Consumption Normal

Our health represents our current standards. By changing your standards when it comes to food – when you eat and what you eat – you will create a domino effect of transformation around the holiday table and your work as well! Next time someone offers to bring something to the next meeting, jump in and volunteer to do the same. Coordinate with others about meal preferences, and don't be surprised if people are totally content with coffee and donuts. The point is to change this, as the latter is an easy and safe go-to for most. Sometimes meetings are scheduled in restaurants, and it's not necessarily up to you to sway the majority. Go back to what I mentioned about deviating from your normal. Deviating once in a while is not the problem; it's the frequency with which we do this: at break, in meetings, during happy hours. You see? It adds up. So, if you're thinking of bringing something delicious and not the typical donut/cookie combo to share with others, check out the recipes below. Happy eating!

MOVE YOUR BODY!

If you are tired, stressed, caught up in deadlines, or find yourself on an emotional rollercoaster, there's no better way to change your physiology and improve your state of well-being than through movement. Grab a co-worker and walk some stairs, or opt for a short walk outside. Our brains are hardwired to make choices that will bring us the most pleasure and minimal pain. For most of us, reaching for a satisfying snack can bring temporary pleasure, never mind the long-term pain and consequences it produces in our bodies. However, when you move your body, you increase the natural endorphin, dopamine, and serotonin production that you would normally get from food, and it becomes the new norm for you, which not only feels good but also produces great results—higher production, cognitive improvement, increased energy, and smaller waistline!

Aside from work and social gatherings, the people closest to us, such as our family members, can have a tremendous impact on our lifestyle and food choices. I am not a clinical psychologist, but as a doctor, I have counseled hundreds of families, couples, and teenagers going off to college and have witnessed many different scenarios around differing food preferences. I have also mentored high school students completing senior projects regarding family nutrition and have helped design recipes that almost everyone can enjoy. There's always someone, however, who will only eat spaghetti in butter sauce, and I have yet to find a cure for that.

As a mom and someone who specializes in nutrition in my private practice, I understand parents who are trying to get their kids to make healthier food choices, and I understand kids, who are not so sure about that. I also understand couples who have differing food preferences and opposing nutritional goals, because it's normal for that to happen. Alignment is sometimes not what we're after.

Whenever I work with families and couples, I first try to understand everyone's baseline: food preferences, eating habits, and also general health. From there we can start a discussion about the impact that certain dietary choices can have on our health and well-being. As a teenage athlete, I struggled with an eating disorder because I simply didn't know what to eat, and I was playing six to nine hours of tennis every day. My mom also didn't know what my needs were, so she sent me to a nutritionist and my own Naturopathic doctor to help me figure it out. The process was not simple and was sometimes challenging considering what my peers were eating for fuel: cookies dipped in milk, soda instead of water, and bagels overflowing with cream cheese.

Having gone through this personal struggle, and also seeing this as a professional, I can tell you that although each situation is unique, the fundamentals of eating wholesome and minimally processed foods never change. The trick is to find what works for most members of the family. It doesn't even have to work all the time to be worthwhile. I truly believe that whole foods are not only good for us but can also taste good. One of my intentions with the recipes that I provide throughout this book is to show how you can take your favorite sweet, salty, and processed snack and find a healthy alternative that others can enjoy as well.

After you have the baseline set for yourself, your family, or your relationship, figuring out why you want to change is the next big step before you start focusing on the what. I'll give you an example of a couple that I had a pleasure of working with.

One of my patients came to me because she was about to get married, and she wanted to be the healthiest version of herself before the big day. She and her fiancé were also talking about having kids, and she wanted to discuss some of her eating and lifestyle habits before she became a mom. As excited as she was to get started, her partner was not on the same page, and it impacted her dramatically. She questioned herself, the future, and even her desire to have a child. This was a perfect time to hear both of their stories.

As it turns out, her fiancé felt that the changes my patient wanted to implement were affecting him, and he was determined to keep the status quo. I applied the principle I shared earlier, establishing a baseline for both of them. When we got a baseline for general health, it was eye-opening for him to see how similar and different their dietary and lifestyle choices were and how unhealthy he really was—his blood sugar was high, he felt tired most mornings, his coffee intake was through the roof, and he had borderline hypertension. His food preferences were fueling some of these findings. He never took the time to question how he ate, slept, moved, and even felt until his partner decided to embark on a journey to better health.

The couple came up with their own individual why's and also a joint why for their desire to get healthy. They both had big career goals and felt that being healthier would help them grow professionally. They both wanted to start a family and wanted to be role models to their kids. Individually, he wanted to feel energized naturally and not rely on stimulants throughout the day, while she just wanted to feel good about herself. Although I could have dug deeper to get to the core of the why, this was enough to keep them on track.

The different environments we weave through during the day can make it challenging for us to make the best choices. However, there are many things we can do to prepare for any situation.

When it comes to family nutrition, I highly recommend Cynthia Lair's *Feeding the Whole Family: Recipes for Babies, Young Children, and Their Parents.* As the title suggests, the book is meant for everyone. Lair provides guidance and instruction on how make any dish kid-friendly, while parents can enjoy a more advanced version. It is simple to follow, ingredients are easy to find, and it is suitable for young foodies and parents alike.

To help you tackle the office space and holiday or social get-togethers, check out the recipes and tips listed at the end of this chapter. They are crowd pleasers easy to prepare and packed with nutrition. Eating healthy, while satisfying your cravings for something decadent, doesn't have to be hard. It just requires a little creativity to find the right food that hits the spot without dire consequences.

►CHAPTER 7 EXERCISES: Recipes for Overcoming Holiday and Office Food Mishaps

Holiday Recipes:

The trick to holiday get-togethers is to 1) not arrive hungry, 2) bring plenty of food that you know you can eat and not feel guilty about, and 3) step away from the cheesecake, ice cream, and triple-layered provocations. Below are a few recipes that are hearty, sweet, crunchy, and tasty enough for everyone to enjoy! Make all three when you're headed to your next party, and bring extra or leave some at home for leftovers.

Colorful, Zesty Carrot and Tahini Salad
Servings: 4-5

So many ways to work this recipe! Have it as a side dish, as an appetizer, as the main dish, or toss it with your favorite green salad. This is a favorite year-round and is easy to make with just a few ingredients.

7 large rainbow carrots

10 ounce can drained chickpeas

1/3 cup olive oil or avocado oil

1/2-1 tsp balsamic vinegar

1 tsp ground turmeric

1/2 tsp paprika

1/2 tsp ginger powder

1/4 tsp garlic salt or sea salt

1/4 tsp pepper

Fresh cilantro

Tahini Dressing:

1/4 cup tahini butter

1/2 Tbsp non-refined apple cider vinegar

1/4 tsp sea salt

1 Tbsp maple syrup or honey

Black pepper to taste

2-3 Tbsp warm nut milk of choice

Optional: 1/4 tsp mustard powder or 1/4 tsp cumin

Preheat oven to 425°F. Rinse and cut carrots into circle shape about .5 cm in thickness.

Drain the canned chickpeas and place in a large bowl with the carrots. Coat with the oil, spices, and balsamic vinegar and lay on a well-greased baking sheet. Roast in the oven for about 30 minutes, turning halfway, and adding more time as necessary depending on firmness. Remove from the oven and toss with salt and pepper. To prepare the dressing, blend Tahini Dressing ingredients in the food processor or blender and adjust sweetness by adding more honey/maple syrup and creaminess/thickness by adding more tahini butter. You can add more vinegar or oil to make the dressing thinner. Plate the carrots, drizzle with the dressing, and serve with chopped cilantro. Keep the dressing in the refrigerator to use with other salads or with leftovers! Enjoy!

Cinnamon Honey Almonds

Servings: 2 cups

This is a great holiday or office party treat. Have these ready to snack on or serve them up for a healthy dessert. Not all sugar is created equal. Honey is a natural sweetener that has a lower glycemic load compared to regular sugar, so it won't spike your blood sugar as quickly, especially when paired with a healthy nut fat. Cinnamon is also a great spice to use, as it helps to reduce sugar consumption. Research has shown that cinnamon can help control blood glucose levels by minimizing insulin spike after meals.[2] (Cinnamon rolls, unfortunately, do not have the same effect.) Dig into this delicious yet awesomely healthy party favorite snack, and tame that sweet tooth while you're at it!

2 cups raw almonds

3 Tbsp raw honey

1/2 tsp of cinnamon

1 tsp sea salt

Preheat oven to 350°F. Place almonds in a bowl. Warm honey to liquefy, pour over the almonds, and mix well so that the almonds are coated evenly. Line a baking sheet with parchment paper, and spread the almond mixture onto it. Sprinkle the nuts with the sea salt and bake for 15-25 minutes, turning occasionally. Allow to cool to room temperature and store in an airtight container. Eat them, give them as gifts, or make everyone happy at the office!

Roll it Up! Zucchini "Sushi"

Servings: 16-20 Rolls

A protein packed snack, meal, or appetizer (depending on how many you have). This is so easy to make, and it is packed with flavor. It is a great alternative to the typical fried, processed, cheesy, or greasy appetizers floating around holiday parties. Hummus can be a great vegetarian source of protein and fat, which is always a plus! I highly recommend alternating different sources of protein to get the most from your nutrition. It's part of eating in a way that is sustainable. Our ancestors did not have access to freezer loads of meat, and in a time when our food supply chain is polluted, resorting to more vegetarian sources of protein is better for the planet and also our health. Cheers!

1 medium zucchini

1 cup garlic hummus or any other hummus

1 cup quinoa, cooked

1/2 cup fresh cilantro

16 leaves fresh basil

1/2 cup finely sliced red pepper

1/2 cup finely sliced carrot, about 2-inch long strips

Lemon, optional

20 toothpicks

Using a mandoline slicer, slice the zucchini lengthwise into thin strips to make about 20 slices, depending on the zucchini. In a mixing bowl, mix the hummus and quinoa. Place 1 tablespoon of the mixture on each zucchini slice and spread it evenly. Place some of the cilantro and basil on one end of the zucchini slice and place pepper and carrots on top. Drizzle with some lemon juice and roll it up! Secure with toothpick. Repeat for the remaining zucchini slices!

Office-Friendly Treats:

I have a sickness. I like doing audits. But not the kind of audits that make you lose sleep at night. I like doing nutrition audits. In fact, I am available for office audits to help you and your office mates have a healthier break room and lunch meetings! Why are we still ordering sandwiches for lunches when we're also sitting at our offices for 12-16 hours a day? It's quick, cheap, and easy, and it's a direct road to excess calories, weight gain, and the desk syndrome, which I would classify as having a host of physical, mental, and emotional symptoms. Next time you plan a meeting, volunteer to make one of the recipes below, and give something to you and your team that will only increase their energy and productivity and make them happy. Who doesn't want to work with happy people? On top of that, if you're having a one-on-one, make it a walk-and-talk meeting. You do enough sitting during the day. Unlike muscle and bone tissue, which gets weaker the less we use it, fat depots in fat cells expand when they experience sustained loading. Research findings affirm that our buttocks not only expand but also stiffen once fat tissue starts to grow in the region, compared with muscle and bone tissue, which wither away when not constantly engaged.[41]

Fudge Bars Reinvented

Servings: 6 bars

Requires a freezer! This recipe has lots to rave about. Loaded with natural sweetness and lots of healthy fats, these bars will give you the lift you need midmorning or afternoon and will satisfy the gnarliest of chocolate cravings. Especially around 2 p.m.

1 cup pitted dates, soaked in water for 1 hour and drained

4 Tbsp raw cacao powder

2 bananas

1 1/2 cup raw almonds.

1/2 cup raw cashews

1/2 cup raw walnuts

1 Tbsp unrefined coconut oil

2 Tbsp raw honey

Place dates, first two tablespoons of cacao powder, cashews, and walnuts in the food processor and mix until well combined. Spread the mixture in a baking pan and press firmly with your fingertips. Mix almonds in the food processor to make texture like almond butter. Pause once in a while and turn the mixture with a spoon. Next add bananas, honey, coconut oil, and the rest of the cacao powder to the almond mixture and process to a smooth paste. Pour the almond, banana, cacao mixture over the date and nut paste in the baking pan and spread evenly. Cover with foil and freeze for 30 minutes. Remove, cut into desired shape, and serve. Don't worry if it softens between home and work, just use a spoon to get all the goodness! Treat it as an ice cream cake, except better!

Carrot Cake Protein Cookies

Servings: 14 cookies

Protein-packed cookies are hard to resist. A great addition to any office meeting, party, or simply whenever. Unlike traditional cookies, these won't make you crash or crave more and are completely made from whole foods that are satisfying and real. Make double and save for later!

1/2 cup creamy nut/seed butter

1 large egg

2 Tbsp melted coconut oil

1/4 cup honey

3 Tbsp unsweetened applesauce or banana

1 tsp vanilla extract

2/3 cup almond meal or almond flour

2 Tbsp coconut flour

1/2 Tbsp ground cinnamon

1 scoop of protein powder of choice

1/2 cup crushed walnut pieces

1/4 cup unsweetened shredded coconut

3/4 cup shredded carrots or apples

In a large mixing bowl, combine nut butter with egg, oil, applesauce or banana, honey, and vanilla extract. Use a kitchen aid, whisk, or blender. Stir in the almond meal or almond flour and the shredded coconut and mix well. Toss in the shredded carrots or apples and put in the fridge for 20 minutes to cool. Preheat oven to 350°F, and line a baking sheet with parchment paper or a silicone mat. Use a tablespoon or cookie scoop to form a cookie on the baking sheet. Leave two inches in between cookies, and flatten the dough into a cookie about two inches wide. Bake for 12-15 minutes until they start to turn a golden color and are not soft in the middle. Allow to cool and transfer to cooling rack. Store in a sealed container in the fridge for optimal freshness.

You can also make more, freeze them, and defrost as needed overnight in the fridge! A great post-lunch snack.

Coconut Snow Balls

Servings: 10

You've probably noticed that many of my recipes have lots of healthy fats. That's because good fat is a power fuel. It gives us the energy we need to conquer the day and the satisfaction that we crave. Maca powder, an herb native to the high Andes of Peru, is an added bonus that is used for overall hormone health and vitality—everything you need to make the most out your day. Grab a dessert/snack like this and get your work on!

1 cup coconut butter or manna

1 cup shredded, unsweetened coconut

3 Tbsp maple syrup or honey

2 tsp pure vanilla extract

Dash of sea salt

1 Tbsp of Maca Powder

1/2 cup more shredded coconut for rolling

Place all ingredients, except the shredded coconut used for rolling, into a food processor and combine until the mixture is smooth and starts forming a ball. Sprinkle the shredded coconut used for rolling onto a baking sheet or large plate. Form small, bite size coconut balls from the prepared dough and roll them in the shredded coconut. Place them onto a baking dish or into a large container and serve right away or store in the fridge to make them firm. You can even freeze them for a frosty treat.

Chapter 8:
The Path to Better Health: Rewiring Our Brain and Cravings

"You can rewire your brain. It's about conditioning. We turn to food on autopilot, and we're eating before we even realize it."

— SUSAN ALBERS

At the root of our decision-making is emotion. In earlier chapters, I discussed many physiological reasons and all sorts of external stimuli that can contribute to cravings. From my experience, if these components are not taken care of, everything else becomes palliative, and results are short-lived. Aside from basic and more complex reasons for why someone craves and chooses processed foods, mindfulness is a hot topic to discuss. From awareness to consciousness and visualization, our minds have the power to influence all aspects of our lives, including personal health and wellness.

The quote by Susan Albers, author of *50 Ways to Soothe Yourself Without Food*, describes a term in psychology known as "cognitive tunneling," also termed as inattentional blindness, which is often the culprit of our decisions around food. Please note that I am using my interpretation of cognitive tunneling in the context of making decisions related to nutrition, as this is not classically how it is used. Nonetheless, when you're at a buffet or roaming the aisles of a grocery store, where does your attention go? Do you channel your focus on the plethora of healthy options or on what will provide instant gratification?

A lot of research has been done in the area of making decisions under stress. Although the brain is capable of performing highly complex tasks and processes an extensive amount of information at any moment in time, under stressful circumstances, it resorts to the easiest decision or action—something that has been practiced before and comes naturally with a snap of the fingers.

In his book *Smarter Faster Better: The Secrets of Being Productive in Life and Business*, Charles Duhigg states that "cognitive tunneling can cause people to become overly focused on whatever is directly in front of their eyes or become preoccupied with immediate tasks. It's what keeps someone glued to their smartphone as the kids wail or pedestrians swerve around them on the sidewalk. It's what causes drivers to slam on their brakes when they see a red light ahead."

Cognitive tunneling has been termed by psychologists for decades. However, the process dates back to the saber-toothed tiger era. It is a protective and purely survivalist mechanism that, unfortunately, does not work as intended in modern times. You can see cognitive tunneling in action multiple times a day as it pertains to our decisions around health.

Let me give you some simple examples of cognitive tunneling and food. In this first example, you're at a grocery store after a twelve-hour work day with whining kids in the shopping cart – or it's the whining voice inside your head reminding you how tired and hungry you are. Even if you are prepared with a shopping list, the stress of being in a store, hungry and tired after a long day, can prompt you to purchase things that you will later regret. That's because in the moment, you seek instant gratification without first checking in to see where the desire is coming from and what the long term ramifications are. Instant gratification – the food is easy to cook, or it tastes good, or you simply deserve it – can be powerful and misleading.

In another example, you're at a dinner with friends, and you're caught off guard as people start ordering food. You haven't made your decision, and the person next to you wants to hear all about you. Enter panic mode, and you order something that you know will taste good and that you've probably had before. You consider this your cheat day, or your second...wait, is it the third day this week? There's absolutely nothing wrong with having a cheat day. But again, it's about the frequency with which you do it. On top of that, many of my clients have experienced negative consequences from cheat days—bloating, fatigue, extra weight, and remorse.

In your own health, where have you seen impulsive behavior become a destructive force?

A patient of mine, who had a very stressful job working as a financial director, would get emotional just talking about her work and the impact it had on her psyche. Her frustration with the direction her career was going, with team dynamics, and with tension at home made it really easy for her to reach for the easy targets: candy, cheese, pasta, jam, and bite size treats. "I get wound up and lose control," she would say. "I know that it's not the best decision, but I just don't care in the moment."

Cultivating awareness is the first step we can take to create long-lasting impact in our health and in our lives. The biggest mistake people make when it comes to nutrition is lack of awareness or mindfulness. We feel and react without giving it further thought until we find ourselves reaching for the cookie jar or finishing a pint of ice cream. This happens not just with food but with other habits and behaviors as well. The exercises you learn in this chapter can easily be applied to other aspects of your life, personal and professional.

Nutrition researchers have studied the correlation between activities like yoga and mindful eating and how skills acquired in the process lead to better dietary and health outcomes. Mindful eating can be looked at as a non-judgmental awareness of physical and emotional sensations while eating, while being in food-related environments, or when you are about to reach for that bag of chips at the checkout line. Because mindful eating can help decrease impulsivity around food, it is exceptionally helpful in decreasing our tendency to react to cravings.

One study in particular developed a tool called the Mindful Eating Questionnaire (MEQ) that compared yoga practitioners to determine if they had higher MEQ scores than non-yoga practitioners and whether lower MEQ scores are associated with body mass index (BMI). It concluded, not surprisingly, that yoga practitioners had higher MEQ scores, but that it did not necessarily translate into lower BMI. It's one thing to be mindful and another to act (or not act) on whatever you're being mindful of.

When I ask my patients to name the number one root cause of their poor eating habits, their equivocal answer is: stress. Stress has the tendency to take any good learned behavior and throw it out the window. Patients will report knowing that what they're doing in times of stress is destructive but having no control over it.

One study noted that, "when you're stressed or unhappy, you may be more inclined to go for sugary foods. This might be due to your taste buds being more receptive to these foods during these times. The tongue contains receptors called glucocorticoids, which are activated during periods of anxiety and stress. They make sweet foods taste even better."[39] This helps explain why it can be so easy to start eating and so hard to stop eating during a stressful experience. This also makes a case for mindfulness and suggests that being more proactive rather than reactive during a stressful situation can lead to fulfillment and better health outcomes.

In regard to my stressed and dissatisfied patient, besides balancing hormones and neurotransmitters, I spent most of our time talking about the different ways she could incorporate mindfulness in her daily routine from family to her workplace. I had her walk stairs several times a day whenever a perceived negative experience was happening. I also helped her balance her blood sugar with a list of healthy go-to snacks that she could have in abundance throughout the day (and that you have access to in this book!). And I asked her to find a breathing or a visualization exercise that helped her get grounded during the day. It only took four visits with a couple more tune ups, and she was in a completely difference space mentally and physically.

Mindfulness is a learned skill that can help generate awareness around cravings and is also a tool for managing cravings. Just as we train our muscles at the gym using weights, we train our minds with mindfulness. Most people believe that mindfulness involves time spent sitting cross-legged, meditating. Although sitting meditation is one way of practicing mindfulness, it is far from the only way. I am a huge proponent of making mindfulness an inseparable part of daily activities. I want to show you how a few different mindfulness practices can be applied in daily life and in managing cravings in particular.

HOW TO MAKE MINDFULNESS A DAILY HABIT

Meditation:

There is no exact number of minutes you need to meditate and no particular position you need to assume. Meditation is about finding a time to settle into your body and breath. You can assume whatever position is comfortable for you—sitting, lying down, or even walking. Your meditation practice can be as short as a few minutes before you head out the door or as long as you want it to be, time permitting. When I find myself pushed for time, I meditate while walking the dog and pushing the stroller, which may seem contradictory, but meditation does not necessarily mean being still in one place. The key with meditation is observation. Although I encourage you to find a time in your day when you can be still and allow your nervous system and body to relax, I also understand the importance of applying the principles of meditation throughout the day.

Whether you are walking, driving, or sitting still, the key is to see your thoughts, emotions, and feelings as transient rather than something permanent that defines you. In relation to food, when you have a craving that is overwhelming, it's a good time to reflect on the source of that craving, such as the emotional state (anger, boredom, sadness etc.) or a triggering event. Where is the sweetness lacking in your life, and what are you trying to compensate for?

Take a moment to breathe through your feelings, knowing that no feeling lasts forever, and allow the cravings to pass rather than acting on them. There are many downloadable phone apps available as well as books and resources on meditation. Find what works best for you, and, most importantly, give it time.

One of my patients was frustrated that meditation did not help her manage stress after just one session. I encouraged her to try to find the best method that would work for her and to try it for at least one month. Sure enough, within a few weeks she noticed dramatic improvement in stress, sleep, and her eating behavior.

Exercise & Movement:

There's no better way to take attention off whatever the mind is preoccupied with than movement, such as exercise, walking, or stretching. Exercise is the most natural way to enhance mood. Multiple studies have shown that exercise, when combined with other therapies, such as meditation and cognitive behavior therapies, helps to decrease symptoms of depression, anxiety, and addictions, such as smoking. If exercise has so many good benefits, including the ability to help manage addictions – in this case, addiction to certain foods – why does 25 percent of the population resort to not doing anything at all? Setting the bar too high may be the case. Focusing on incorporating movement throughout the day rather than for some set time is much more sustainable and suitable for most individuals.[19] When you take an extra walk during the day, do a short core exercise in the morning, or simply go for a jog around the block, you are changing your physiology, which, in turn, changes how you feel.

To earn my degree, I had to be in school for twelve years. That's a lot of books, exams, and sitting. I am grateful that my parents had instilled in me the importance of an active lifestyle early on. I carried that through my whole life. So even when I was pursuing a business degree and then a doctorate in Naturopathic Medicine, I didn't skip a beat, and I also didn't gain a pound. I joke that during exams, I was in peak shape because for every hour of studying, I would do ten minutes of exercise. I'm a huge believer in the idea that you don't need an hour a day of dedicated gym time. Make it a part of your daily life, just as with meditation. Challenging yourself to start your day with a short workout of your choice, walking stairs during lunch, and going for a bike ride in the evening (or whatever else you want to do!) will make the biggest difference in your life. You will find that you also lean toward healthier food choices, as movement brings clarity.

If you're still convinced that you don't have ten minutes for yourself because of kids, job, or anything else, I don't believe that talk, and neither should you! Health is the number one priority. Without health, our goals become much less appealing and even less achievable. I was in for a reality check when my son was born, as most parents are with their first child. For the first maybe ten months, my morning and evening routines were gone, I didn't have an hour each day to exercise or train, and I was running a medical practice and a business. However, I did have ten minutes I could scavenge during the day, and I aimed to get longer workouts in on the weekends whenever I could. Slowly the scavenging for time actually turned into a routine. Looking at my day the night before, I knew exactly when and where I could squeeze in a quick weight session, a yoga sequence, a brisk walk, or even a short jog. But it is all because I prioritized my day around movement, as it is vital to my health and performance on many levels.

So go ahead; get your move on!

Meal Time:

Practicing mindfulness while eating is one of the best ways to experience fulfillment when it comes to food, and it also helps us become aware of our relationship to food. Most of us inhale food during a meal or work through our lunches and dinners. The amount of work we need to process during a workday and the pressure to finish is high, so it's understandable that you need to squeeze every minute out of the day. I am guilty of this as well, and it's also something I am working on. But it's still important to make a point to have your meals away from the work desk.

Taking the time to chew, smell, and experience the joy of having a meal will help with digestion and the absorption of nutrients. It will also make you feel more full, as it takes thirty minutes to experience the feelings of satiety after a meal. So the longer you take to eat your meal, the more likely it is that the feeling of satisfaction will hit right as your meal is done. Being mindful of what's on your plate is also a key to understanding why you may be craving something sweet or salty after a meal. Reaching for something that looks good is a subconscious decision. Choosing to have a balanced meal with lean protein and a balance of healthy carbohydrates and fat is a conscious decision.

I rarely go to a hot food bar at my local store without knowing what I'll get, and I rarely arrive at a restaurant without first looking at the menu. Plan to succeed by being mindful not only when you're eating but also before you get to your meal. There's a good reason why meal planning is popular. It helps you stay focused on what it is you need when the hangry voice inside starts crying for something else.

A study involving smokers solidifies what happens in the brain during a craving and compares with the relationship between mindfulness, mindful eating, and cravings. The study recruited forty-seven smokers who wanted to quit and asked them to abstain from smoking for twelve hours before the experiment was conducted. Researchers taught the participants basic principles of mindful attention, a simple intervention that required no formal meditation training. Researchers showed the smokers smoking-related images designed to induce cravings.

The smokers were asked to view some of the images passively, without any special mindfulness. They were asked to view other images mindfully. In the process, the researchers asked the smokers to report any cravings they were experiencing. At the same time, using a functional magnetic resonance image machine, researchers watched what was happening in each smoker's brain, tracking brain activity.

It turned out that mindfulness reduced cravings, which is actually counter-intuitive because previous research has shown that images trigger strong cravings in smokers. Mindfulness, however, seems to provide some kind of immunization to the images. In addition, reduced cravings correlated with reduced activity in craving-related areas of the brain, also known as the anterior cingulate cortex. What's more, mindfulness didn't just reduce activity, it disconnected the different regions of the brain that make up the craving network of neural connections.[20]

To apply this to food cravings, paying mindful attention to the trigger of the craving can interrupt this complex brain response, build new neural connections and behaviors, and ultimately protect people from their own desire to give into the temptation—which is a constant work in progress. My clients always ask me if overriding the impulsive habits surrounding cravings ever gets easier, and the answer is YES! But it requires your personal commitment to health, the desire to change your environment, mindfulness, and long term vision for yourself.

I want to conclude this chapter with an exercise to stimulate your personal vision for your health using a hands-on visualization technique. Too many of us fall off the bandwagon because we don't remember why we're doing something in the first place. I hope the information provided in this book will not only help you get to the root cause of cravings but will also provide value in other areas of your life.

Visualization is a highly effective technique that has been used in psychology to help people achieve greater personal and professional outcomes. It combines mindfulness with intention and is a great tool for overriding impulsive behavior. Research has shown that food cravings target the same parts of the brain that are used in basic cognitive tasks. Visualization and memory-engaging activities, such as thinking of a pleasurable activity, have been shown to reduce cravings for food.[52] Although more research needs to be done to assess the long term efficacy of visualization techniques on cravings, visualization is definitely an exercise to consider incorporating into your daily flow.

There are many different ways to use visualization. One of my favorite activities is creating a vision board. Because visualization has the power to change how we experience cravings, rather than thinking about which image you want to substitute for the nagging craving, create a vision board to help you choose images that you can easily remember and that you've developed strong feelings for. Vision boards are one of many ways to bring visualization to life.

Jump into this next creative section, and start cultivating a vision for a healthy you, craving free! If you're a skeptic, I'll explain the physics behind this exercise.

►CHAPTER 8 EXERCISES: Create Your Perfect Health Vision Board—Bringing Your Vision into Reality

"The law of attraction is forming your entire life experience and it is doing that through your thoughts."
—THE SECRET

Visualization is one of the most powerful tools and exercises you can use to realize your goals, and it is available to everyone. Professional athletes have used visualization for years to improve performance. Research shows that brain patterns activated during an activity are also activated when the activity is visualized.[3]

In this section, I'll show you how to transform your vision for yourself into reality and how to create the life you want to live.

A vision board is a great way to transform how you want to feel and what you want to achieve into visual form. It also channels your attention toward what you want rather than what you don't want. "Like attracts like" is a big component to all of this and is best explained by the concept of "strong interaction" or "strong force" from quantum physics.

On a fundamental level, everything is made of atoms, and atoms are made of the building blocks of neutrons, protons, and electrons with the nucleus in the center. The nucleus is made of protons and neutrons. Normally, protons, being of the same charge, would repel each other. But the nucleus is held together by the strong force or, in this case, nuclear force. The nuclear force that keeps the protons together is by far stronger than any other force.

In 1935, Dr. Hideki Yukawa, a Nobel prize physicist, discovered that neutrons and protons in the nucleus of the atom constantly emit "virtual particles" called mesons. The exchange of these mesons among the subatomic particles is the strong force that holds the nucleus of the atom and physical reality together.

Our thoughts, our feelings, and everything else for that matter are composed of energy, such as the energy of light, and are, therefore, governed by quantum physics. The same principles that apply to protons and neutrons apply to our thoughts.[4]

The difference between everything else and our thoughts is that we have the ability to regulate our thoughts, train our mind, and make conscious decisions.

Peter Baksa, the author of The Point of Power, states that "our minds are transceivers, able to receive and send signals into the 'quantum soup' by way of the highly coherent frequencies of our thoughts."[53] As we think, so we become, as the saying goes.

Beyond thoughts, there are feelings. Tony Robbins, the guru of transformation, talks a lot about transforming your state by changing simply how you feel. So the big question to ask in transitioning into the next section is: How do you want to feel?

As you make your vision board, think about the possible feelings you want to experience on your journey to better health and a crave free life. Do you want feelings of liberation, happiness, and fulfillment, or maybe joy, satisfaction, and vitality?

To start your vision board, first identify the feelings that you want to experience, and then choose images or items you've collected, which you can put on your vision board and which will bring you closer to your vision. On my vision board, I have lots of pictures of the great outdoors, my family, and also affirmations for how I want to feel and experience life. Because there are certain foods that I want to see more of in my life, as they make me feel amazing, I have pictures of nourishing salads, vegetable gardens, and words of affirmation such "healthy mind and body."

My board is strategically placed in our master bedroom so that as I walk in and out, I come face to face with the reminder of what it is that I seek to experience and realize. When I take a moment to pause during the day, I recall the images on the vision board to help me realign with the feelings I want to experience and my purpose. Like muscles, mindfulness and visualization techniques need to be trained to be effective. Make it a habit to connect with your vision on a daily basis, assign feelings to the images you've selected, and recall these images during times of stress, during afternoon slumps, when you're stuck in traffic, and when certain thoughts regarding cravings for food or other substances start to creep in. Visualization, combined with other techniques mentioned, will absolutely break that negative loop.

If you already have a vision board, see if you can give it a face lift. Your vision board should bridge the gap between where you are now and where you want to be. By addressing the psychology of cravings, you become an unstoppable force moving toward your true purpose and potential.

Chapter 9
Staying the Course

"Difficult times disrupt your conventional ways of thinking and push you to forge better habits of thought, performance, and being."

—Robin Sharma

My first experience with a cleanse was when I was about fifteen years old. My mom and my older sister were into that sort of thing, so of course, I wanted to be just like them. I would juice, sweat in the sauna, do water fasts, and even drink olive oil to facilitate liver toxin elimination—which I would not recommend for anyone! Never mind that a fifteen-year-old should not do a cleanse, but on these cleanses, I felt deprived, irritated, and tormented by a great desire to overindulge afterward.

There is yet to be a short-term fix that produces long-term results. I am a fan of the 14-, 30-, 60-day or whatever the magic number is for a cleanse, a detox, or a fitness challenge to reset the body and start new. However, I am even a greater fan of change that extends beyond that. I am talking about change that lasts.

The problem with any program is that it rarely creates long-term change, and this is why summer after summer, people rush to do a challenge of some sort to get their bikini body back, only to undo the work over Thanksgiving dinner. We've all been there, and I am on a mission to end this and create lifelong, sustainable habits.

I get involved in many challenges in my fitness community, in part because I like to provide a key education component, which is life after the challenge. How should you ease back from a challenge into a normal way of eating, exercising, and living? What is that new normal? How do you know what to include or exclude? What happens when things don't go as you expect, plan, or hope for?

I've always felt great just from eating a well-balanced diet along the lines of Michael Pollan's idea to "eat food, not too much, mostly plants," and also following a disciplined workout schedule with lots of variety. My lifestyle worked for me. I would go through very stressful periods in my life and still come out healthier than ever on the other side. That was until I faced a bigger challenge than I had anticipated, which was becoming a mom.

Seven months after delivering our first child, I went through a phase in which no matter what I ate or how much I moved or slept, I kept feeling tired, I was losing hair, and I was finding it harder to stick to my bulletproof dietary habits. The very things that I preached about were not working out for me.

When given just the essential building blocks for good health, like nutritious food and optimal lifestyle habits, the body can function like a well-oiled machine. Every second of the day, on the physiological level, the body is trying to keep things from going astray. Various biochemical processes regulate pH of the blood, maintain body temperature and blood pressure, and control blood sugar, to name just a few. On a cellular level, the cells are receiving messages from hormones and other chemical messengers to perform their specific duty, depending on the type of cell.

Given the right amount of stress, the body does just fine. It adjusts and adapts, and life goes on. Sometimes, however, the amount of stress that someone experiences, either in a moment or over a prolonged period of time, exceeds the body's ability to cope. This can result in a domino effect of a system breakdown.

Think of the body as a stove top. When it's working well, you can cook, doing whatever you need to do to utilize the ingredients.

If it's broken, there are few things you can do, and your options for utilizing those ingredients are limited. For me personally – and many parents can relate – after seven months of waking every hour during the night to care for our baby, working as a doctor, running a business and a medical practice, and being an active member in the community, my body reached its threshold, and my stove top shut down on me.

I knew how to fuel properly, how much to exercise, which foods to increase or to decrease, which supplements to take, and how much sleep to get. The problem was that none of these things mattered in the context of an underlying hormone and nutrient imbalance. This is exactly what I see in my practice every single day. The same information that I share in this book about hormones, neurotransmitters, and nutrition and the recipes to help curb cravings to improve mood, endocrine health, and digestion, are the same principles that I teach my clients and that I had to go through myself.

STAYING THE COURSE STEP #1:

By now you are well aware that food cravings can be a symptom of something bigger. The first step in staying the course is to make sure that you don't have any underlying health conditions. I had a client come in complaining that she was feeling tired and overweight. She mentioned that her go-to was dark chocolate with coffee and different forms of sweets throughout the day, which kept her awake for short periods of time. She was losing hair and gaining weight around the abdomen, and no amount of rest could curb her fatigue.

She mentioned that she had read somewhere that cravings for chocolate could be attributed to a magnesium deficiency, so she started to take magnesium, but she saw little to no improvement in her symptoms. After doing a thorough workup, we identified that she was very low on iron, and she had an underlying thyroid disorder that she was not aware of. Her cravings for chocolate, along with the other symptoms, were part of a much bigger problem that we needed to address in order for her to regain vitality, start losing weight, stop cravings sweets, and improve her productivity naturally.

Another patient of mine was a high-level executive in a top software company. He came in looking to get tips on his diet to help him lose weight. He mentioned that, aside from walking and doing his physical therapy exercises, he didn't have time to exercise, as he was working sixty-hour weeks and juggling parenthood. Most of my patients come to see me after they've already been to nutritionists, their primary care doctor, and other specialists. Simply giving someone nutrition tips for weight loss is rarely part of my strategy, as I like to dig deeper.

In this case, my patient's diet was flawless, and he was doing enough activity that his weight should have been normal. Because the normal range for many lab values, including thyroid, is so big, many providers miss this, as I have mentioned earlier. They are looking for a zebra rather than listening to the patient. My patient's thyroid values were subpar, and his symptoms were reflecting just that. When I helped him improve his thyroid function naturally with very little intervention, he was able to sleep better, lose weight, and experience a higher level of energy amid a crazy schedule. The list of patient stories similar to these that I could share is vast.

STAYING THE COURSE STEP #2:

After ruling out any preexisting health conditions, the second step in staying the course is not to say "screw it" when things don't go the way you planned. I've had many patients say, "No matter what I do, I still gain weight, so I stop caring how I eat." I understand how frustrating it can be, especially when you've been trying to change your health for years. But there are a couple of things that are wrong with this logic and can backfire in the long run.

First, weight is a representation of many factors, and having a well-balanced diet is key whether your weight is shifting or not. You want to set yourself up for success when it comes to health rather than get a host of other health issues, such as elevated blood sugar, increased inflammation, joint pain, and digestive disorders, to list just a few, all of which can be linked to poor nutrition.

Second, most weight issues have an underlying endocrine or hormone problem, as we saw in the earlier chapter about hormones. When that is taken care of, having sustainable dietary and lifestyle habits in place will be the key to keeping weight off. We all know someone who has regained all of their weight back after successful weight loss. This chapter is about making sure that all the bases are covered so you can create life changing and sustaining habits in a healthy body.

Time and time again, I see stories of success and failure. One of my patients had successfully completed a weight-loss program but appeared in my office frustrated that she had regained most of the weight back. "I see the weight creeping back up. It makes me think nothing is working, and everything becomes fair game to me," she said.

I can empathize with the desire to just say, "Screw it." When I was not feeling my optimal by far, it started to impact all aspects of my life—my relationship with my husband, my performance at work, and the most sacred role of all, motherhood. I was trying so hard to eat well, exercise, sleep, and take the right supplements that at many points, I just felt like giving up. Driving to get a slice of pizza sounded a lot more pleasing than taking a stroll outside, and I don't even like pizza.

What kept me going was inherently and deeply knowing that I could not just let things go—it wasn't my style, and far too many people were seeking my advice in similar situations. But I also knew, given my profession as a Naturopathic Physician, that there were many things I could do differently and many biological markers I could look at to see what was going on. Naturopathic medicine is functional medicine, as it looks at all aspects of health and considers the whole person rather than just symptoms. So as much as you many want to say, "Screw it," know that there are many things to consider before giving up.

STAYING THE COURSE STEP #3:

The third step in staying the course is inspired by the book called *Turning Pro* by Steven Pressfield. I learned about Steven and his book when I was doing one of my morning rituals, which is listening to one of the most amazing female entrepreneurs, Marie Forleo, who just happens to have some of the best speakers on her online TV show, Marie TV.

Steven talks about daily habits and behaviors that differentiate amateurs from professionals and tells how to make the switch in our lives to be more like the pros to achieve the results that we want in personal and professional life. You don't have to be a sports fanatic to make it relevant. Think of any area of your life, including your health, where you are making amateur moves that lead to unsatisfactory results. Do you stick to any particular diet plan only to give up on it a week or a month later? Granted, it might not be sustainable, and that's one reason you give it up, but do you actively look for alternatives?

The difference between an amateur and a professional is that the professional, day in and day out regardless of circumstances, strives to perform at a peak level. This can be said about a professional athlete or anyone who is performing at their peak in any industry, profession, or personal life. The habits of top performers are similar to those of professional athletes. They have vision and values, they know their why, and they have the discipline and focus to follow through. They also have the emotional muscle trained to override negative thinking. Mental toughness, fortitude, and motivation are skills that are trained, not necessarily something you have to be born with. You earn these skills through daily practice, and there are many opportunities during the day.

How does this apply to the many aspects of health?

Your desirable state of health is completely up to you. You decide how you want to feel, how much energy you want to have, how happy you want to be, the level of activity you want to have, how you want to look, the quality of life you want to have, and the relationship you want to have with yourself and others. Certain events and unforeseen circumstances happen, or maybe you find yourself in a place where access to health is not as accessible as it is at home. But in the grand scheme of things, it is your decision, your desire, and most importantly, your action!

If you want to improve any aspect of your health, are you searching for solutions and are you implementing them? When you are presented with solutions, does a part of you shy away and give excuses for why they may not work? Do you try a new strategy for a short period of time only to give up on it and go back to old habits? How do you address obstacles to health?

Having a vision in place, a pro does everything in his or her power to get to the goal. It may mean getting up in the morning before everyone else does. It may mean learning new skills and becoming resourceful. It also may mean that you have to surround yourself with the right people and maybe reevaluate your current hierarchy of relationships.

If you seek long-lasting change, change your behavior to match that of the pros, and stop making amateur moves when it comes to your health – and, in fact, any other area of your life.

STAYING THE COURSE STEP #4:

The fourth step in staying the course involves getting rid of habits that no longer serve you. I bet that, off the top of your head, you already know of a couple of habits that need to go. Habits come in pairs, and once in a while, we need to do a habit audit. This is by far one of the hardest things to do, because our habits shape us and our choices and create comfort zones from which it's hard to break free. Some common negative habits that come in pairs include coffee and sugar, alcohol and cigarettes, eating while working, and others that may be more applicable or relevant to you.

Finding alternative habit pairs can be life-changing on multiple levels, including breaking a sugar addiction to improve your health and daily performance. In my personal journey to living a life free of processed foods and sugar, I identified triggers and behaviors throughout the day that fueled my habits around sugar. Then slowly, one trigger at a time, I developed a mindfulness practice similar to the one I've already shared. I also found alternative habits or behaviors to bring about positive change in my life. In my private practice, aside from correcting the underlying imbalances mentioned in this book, I've also helped patients make shifts similar to the ones told in the stories dispersed throughout these chapters.

Most of our heavily imbedded behaviors are driven by the primitive fight or flight response. Except in primitive times, the danger was real. The fight or flight response was necessary and usually involved running away or defending oneself. Nowadays when we experience stress, the fight or flight response kicks in, and we seek out whatever will make us feel comforted and secure— usually in the form of food or other pleasurable activity/distraction.

One person I follow closely is Brendon Burchard, author of *High Performance Habits*. In an interview discussing his book, Brendon mentioned that motivation helps us get to where we want to be, but habits are what help us stay there. He also mentioned a very significant and life-changing concept: achievement does not equal alignment. This is applicable on so many levels when it comes to improving your health and making change that lasts. Let's dig in for a moment.

One reason we keep resorting to old behaviors is because we fail to change our daily habits. How many times have you done a 14-day cleanse only to go back to destructive eating habits on day fifteen? I see this happen all the time. During the 14-day cleanse, you meal prep, you are conscious about what you're eating, you eliminate processed foods, and you focus on healthy eating. Somehow, once the 14 days are up, all the good habits you developed go out the door, and you no longer have the time nor the desire to continue with the program.

If you maintain the healthy habits you developed during the 14 days for a year, five years, or even a lifetime, that's when change happens. But these habits need to be in alignment with who you are and where you want to be. You may start on a health journey for personal reasons—to improve your health, to change relationships around you, or maybe to improve focus and performance. Whatever your reasons are, make sure they align with what you want. It's rare that someone picks up a book or starts a new program when they are completely satisfied with the status quo.

On the journey to better health, there will be times when you fall off the health bandwagon. Family will visit, a business trip will come up, and you will find yourself in a restaurant or at a party where they don't have foods you normally rely on. Honoring the journey and allowing yourself to have a bad day is the next important step in staying the course.

One of my clients, a highly successful woman working in IT sales, had a hard time sticking to her meal plans and eating well, as she traveled all over the country on a weekly basis. She would come back frustrated that on her trip she couldn't find anything to eat, lunch meetings were only sandwiches, and her frustration had led her to make further poor decisions around food. One bad day would lead her to have a bad week and even a bad month. We worked together to correct nutritional deficiencies and hormone imbalances, and I suggested food alternatives given her busy schedule. As a result, she was able to lose over twenty pounds over the course of one year. Still, she was frustrated about not being able to make the best decisions around food one hundred percent of the time. I redirected her attention to show her just how well she was doing and shifted her focus to the things she could control most of the time, even in the most unfavorable situations.

Changing expectations, adapting, and allowing life to happen are part of the journey to better health. The journey requires patience, creativity, and the ability to tweak your health plan. Once in a while, circumstances will challenge whatever you're doing. Your health and personal health goals require the same amount of focus, dedication, and commitment as any other area of your life. Even though many people know this, most still struggle to stay motivated. Take New Year's resolutions for example. If you keep making the same resolutions year after year, you need to do something drastically different.

Over the years, to help patients and clients stay the course, I've led groups of individuals who are motivated to change through what I called "Achieving Personal Health Breakthrough." This was a group setting where we addressed five main topics over the course of several months. People could participate from afar using an online platform, and the group setting provided participants with an opportunity to ask questions, hear what other people had to say, and, most importantly, get the support they needed.

The **first step** in achieving personal health breakthrough is about getting real with yourself. That is called doing a "self-assessment," which is about understanding your current self-talk, owning your story, and facing your weaknesses; realizing that everyone struggles on some level, regardless of their background; and seeing how your current mindset impacts physiology and the actions you take. The most important aspect of doing a self-assessment is recognizing that change will happen when you determine a new standard for yourself.

The moment you decide on a new standard for yourself, without skipping a beat, you need to have your WHY ready. This is the **second step** in the process, because when you want to quit, when you're not fitting in the clothes you want, or you had a bad day, your WHY will remind you of the reason you need to stay the course. Everyone has their own WHY. For some, it can be as simple as wanting to look a certain way, while others may set a new standard so that they can be a better spouse, parent, or friend. Regardless of the reason, it needs to resonate with you, as everyone is motivated by different things.

Committing to your new standard, defining what commitment means to you, and being reasonable is the **third step** of the program. Define what success means to you and work up to it. If your goal is to hit the gym five days a week for an hour, start by going two to three times a week. Hitting it hard from the start will result in a low compliance rate, which means you're more likely to quit after week one.

One of my clients went from living a sedentary lifestyle to signing up for a five-days-a-week 5 a.m. boot camp. As a result, her low back and knees hurt, she was sleep deprived, and she became frustrated very quickly. Had she eased into the process, this could have been avoided. Giving her body a chance to adapt would have yielded better results. Instead, this was like shock therapy. Going from zero to full force is a huge stress on the body, which elevates cortisol levels. If you remember from the chapter on hormone health, cortisol is our fight or flight stress hormone, and no way will your body lose weight in this state!

The **third step** is super important, as there is such a thing as over-commitment, which can result in unnecessary stress and contribute to a vicious cycle of stress, disappointment, and giving up. Avoid this by being clear about what is reasonable for you— not for your friends, neighbors, or co-workers. This is absolutely related to good nutrition. You won't be perfect the first time, the first week or month or maybe even year. Slipups will happen, but know that over time, they will happen less frequently. You'll have an easier time avoiding them by developing your personal tool box of recipes, go-to foods, mindfulness practices, supplements, and the right people to help you stay the course.

Most of us have heard the saying that our habits and behaviors are shaped by the five people closest to us, and to stay the course, this cannot be ignored. Think about it. If you are looking to create long-lasting change in your diet, exercise, career, relationships, finances, or whatever else it may be, who are the people who are influencing your choices in these areas?

My boot camp client brings us to the **fourth step**, which is accountability and consistency. Although she had good intentions to lose weight and live a healthy lifestyle, none of her friends were fit, they all partied together on the weekends, and she was able to find every excuse possible for her slipups. To this day, unfortunately, she has not been able to lose the weight, continues to fuel her negative behaviors, and at the same time wonders why her health is not on track.

Get someone to be your accountability partner, or brainstorm what accountability looks like to you. Some of my clients have found accountability partners through fitness classes, church, or work. Others have reached out to friends and have even formed their own groups. Set a schedule and commit to a weekly or biweekly meeting or phone chat to check in with your partner. We are less likely to falter when we know someone else is watching, and although I'd like the accountability to come from within, I know it's nice when someone else has got your back.

One the most important parts of achieving your personal health breakthrough is to make it sustainable, which is the **fifth step.** This is related to setting realistic expectations, defining your commitment, and also finding a plan or program that you can stick to long-term. One reason I don't like typical cleanses or short-term programs is that once you're done, you're not sure what do. What do you continue to include or exclude? How can you get back on track if you get blindsided by family visits, holidays, or summer vacations?

Because I am a cheerleader for sustainability, having done this myself and helped thousands of people do the same, I've created my own version of a cleanse that is meant to extend beyond its intended timeframe so that you can continue eating in a way that promotes physical, mental, and emotional health without the yo-yo effect. You can find the 14-Day Crave Reset™ Sugar Cleanse at the end of this book along with crave friendly, taste bud approved, and satisfying recipes.

As this chapter concludes, I'd like to reiterate that what we do on a daily basis shapes our habits, our behaviors, and ultimately our health. Focus on what you can do now to make a positive difference in your life, and stick with it by making the necessary changes. Remember, you don't have to have all the answers at once; this is a journey. My greatest hope is that you can walk away with tools and knowledge to help you navigate the path to better health.

The end of this chapter includes time-tested nutrition tips to help you successfully stay the course, as well as a list of things you can do on a daily basis after any challenge or cleanse or as part of your daily health routine!

►CHAPTER 9 EXERCISES: Nutrition Tips and Daily Health Hacks for Long Term Success

Don't skip meals—The longer you go without a meal or snack, the more likely it is that you'll binge, make a bad decision, or overeat. Keeping your blood sugar stable through – and after – any program you decide to pursue will be **key to long term success.**

Stay hydrated—especially when you are doing any sort of detox or cleanse or when you're putting your body through a lifestyle change. Removal of toxins requires hydration. Keep a water bottle with you and refill as needed! Include electrolytes, as well, to keep fluid/electrolyte balance in the body.

Be prepared—Keep a snack in your purse, in your car, at your work desk, in your gym bag—wherever you are! This may sound ridiculous, but the reality is that **when you fail to plan, you plan to fail!**

Balance blood sugar—Aim to combine certain foods for optimal blood sugar balance: **combine protein and fat with a balance of carbohydrates in snacks AND meals.** This combination will slow digestion and increase satiety and won't leave you feeling deprived!

Fuel Optimally—Eat thirty minutes before and within thirty minutes after working out to improve recovery, energy, and performance.

Notice your triggers, and know thyself—Are you hungry OR are you frustrated, upset, or angry? Emotional hunger can be misleading and can leave you with an empty bag of candy or chips in a matter of seconds.

Cultivating Change That Lasts, Daily:

We've all been guilty of trying a new diet or fitness routine, only to watch it slowly disappear out of our lives. After you complete any cleanse or challenge, the main objective is to maintain the good habits you cultivated. The goal is to keep feeling good, so I'd like to share some tips on how to make long-lasting change to your nutrition plan without the emotional and physical roller coaster of dieting.

Start by asking yourself what worked and what didn't during any particular challenge that you've done. What did you find the most challenging, and what surprised you that maybe wasn't as challenging as you anticipated? What are the top three things you could walk away with and make part of your daily eating and moving routine?

We live in a time when we go from one thing to another either without being fully engaged or having no time to reflect. Take a moment to answer these few questions, as they will provide insight into what works best for you and what you can do to keep yourself on course. I've received a lot of feedback over the years regarding my 14-Day Crave Reset™ Sugar Cleanse, which is included at the end of this book. Some of my clients loved the idea of keeping breakfast and dinner simple two days out of the week by having a nourishing smoothie or a protein shake, as it was a no brainer for them. They didn't have to cook, but more important, they felt that these lighter days made them feel more energetic while helping them maintain their wellness and weight goals. They also used these days as opportunities to reset from the weekend or a dinner party or work trip. See if this is something that could work for you. Again, the cleanse is located at the end of this book with the recipes.

After doing something like the 14-Day Crave Reset™ Sugar Cleanse, there are five basic steps you can implement on a daily basis to not only help you cleanse from sugar and processed foods but to also help your organs, like the liver and the gut, remove daily metabolic waste:

1. Always eliminate foods you're sensitive or allergic to. The common culprits are dairy, gluten, soy, corn, citrus, coffee, sugar, and the nightshade family (tomatoes, bell peppers, cayenne pepper, eggplant, white potatoes).

2. Start your morning with a pH balancing tonic. Apple cider vinegar (ACV) is well known for its pH balancing properties. It also improves digestion and liver function. A great morning tonic includes: 1 tsp ACV, 1 tsp maple syrup, 1 tsp lemon juice, 6 oz warm water. Drink upon rising. NOTE: If you are taking thyroid medication, drink thirty minutes after you take the medication.

3. Hydrate, hydrate, hydrate. Water moves waste out of the cellular environment into lymph, and the lymph system clears it out for excretion.

4. Sweat daily. Our biggest organ for eliminating toxins is our skin! Sweating is one of the most optimal and safe ways to eliminate toxins. Sweating protocols are even recommended when eliminating metals, due to safety as opposed to other procedures. Break a sweat with your favorite exercise!

5. Include a liquid fast day **during the week** or **every fourteen days**. I don't recommend water fasts as they are very challenging for people to stick to or to even look forward

to. They can also do more harm if you've got a blood sugar problem, high or low. For this and many other reasons, I recommend a liquid fast with liquids besides water. Here's how I suggest to do a fasting day: In the morning, have a protein shake of your choice. During the day have two 16 oz. fresh squeezed juices with mostly greens and cucumbers and one choice of fruit. Finish the day with another protein shake.

Chapter 10
Food and Performance—
The Direct Link

"I have learned that champions aren't just born; champions can be made
when they embrace and commit to life-changing positive habits"

—LEWIS HOWES

Everyone has their personal why or reason for wanting to tame their food cravings and create healthier eating habits. For some, addressing a food craving is a matter of achieving better health. For others, the craving is about weight loss and changing habits in other areas of life. The types of foods we choose to consume and fuel our bodies with, however, extends beyond weight loss and physical health. I am talking about the next level of optimal health, which is peak performance.

Performance can have multiple meanings, depending on who you are and what meaning you associate with it. If you are a professional athlete, your definition of performance and what you do to achieve it is different from but similar to a busy professional working fifty-plus hour weeks and taking care of a family. Regardless of the profession or title, everyone needs to perform. The foundation of excellent performance is great nutrition, because with great nutrition comes health, and when you're healthy, anything is possible.

In my private practice, I see athletes, weekend warriors, full-time parents, top level executives, board members, and busy professionals climbing the corporate ladder. All of them have the need to excel and achieve peak performance given the mental and physical stressors of the day. They may not make that link initially, but that changes quickly. Athletes and non-athletes alike have the same stress response, which is simply different in its magnitude but similar in the physiological outcome.

Fundamentally, there are things that we can control when circumstances and events are not exactly favorable. You hear many leaders in performance coaching and education (such as Tony Robbins, Tim Ferriss, Marie Forleo, Gabby Bernstein, Tom Bilyeu, Lewis Howes, and Ryan Holiday, to name just a few) talk about the importance of our mental and physiological state and how to change it to achieve our desired outcomes (in a nutshell). I'd like to add that when you pay attention to what you put in your body, when you understand the different factors that affect the absorption and metabolism of nutrients, and when you can correct whatever is getting in the way of your peak health—you are more likely to succeed and follow through with personal and professional goals. Allow me to elaborate a bit more and mention that your psychology is absolutely key to your success and daily performance, but it works only as long as you have healthy physiology. Otherwise, it's like putting a pretty veneer on a decayed tooth. It looks fine and seems fine, but eventually you need to address a deeper problem that will cause issues in the long run.

One reason food cravings are important to address in terms of performance is that food has become a distraction for many people. It makes sense why—you only have to go back to earlier chapters and revisit the biochemical pathways to see that certain foods are addicting, like some very potent drugs. Instead of using food as medicine, we medicate with food. We're happy, we eat. We're sad, we eat. We're angry, why not, let's eat. The list of reasons to eat is endless.

No one is immune to this, and everyone has their struggle, but the stories are similar. I have elite athletes complaining about their sugar problem and employees dismayed with their constant sugar runs throughout the day. Then there's the end of the day, when you get home after a long day of slaying emails and meetings, and your one wish is to plop on the couch and indulge in a decadency of some sort. I see and hear this all the time, and I train people to overcome the desire to just crash. I help people improve their physiology and psychology so that they have the energy to start and finish their day strong, and I always loop back to nutrition as the cornerstone of peak performance.

Aside from our mood and emotions fueling our cravings and distracting us from our day-to-day goals and activities, the changing work environment contributes to this issue as well. More companies are switching to open work spaces and working from home, which makes food even a greater distraction. According to an article from Fast Company titled, "The 10 Worst Things About Working in an Open-Office–In Your Words," food smells made it to the top ten list. Even if you're not ready for a meal, your buddy next door is, and whatever they are eating fuels your senses and appetite.

In further research, the media organization People Matter, which focuses on human resources, concluded from a survey that food is definitely one of the bigger distractions—particularly in regard to what other people are eating, as well as eating at the desk. Essentially, other people's food choices effect your food preferences and also the timing of your meals, which makes it even more important to develop healthy habits around food and to stick to them regardless of what your colleagues are doing. Otherwise you are following someone's else's cues and not your own!

In another example, *Globe And Mail* found that companies like CBRE, a commercial real estate service company, have gone as far as to limit eating at the work desk. The company discovered that the new policy encouraged employees to socialize more, keep their work desks clean, and stay focused on the task at hand. The overall effect was that more work got done with less stress. Amazing what can happen when you make a simple change that results in greater health outcomes, such as decreased stress and increased productivity. This should be part of any company culture and not just policy, because policy means something needs to be enforced, but when we talk about something being part of a company's culture, then we start getting into values and beliefs rather than just rules.

What about the folks who work from home and are not directly involved in the company culture?

Jane Heminsley, in her article for *The Guardian* titled "Avoiding the Distractions of Working from Home," summed it up beautifully: "It's true that little routines do give structure to your working from home schedule, but take care not to fall into the trap of using the kettle as a crutch in every situation. Tricky call with a client? That was awkward, I'll make myself a cuppa to recover. Land a new contract? Coffee and biscuits to celebrate. Not quite sure where this piece of work is going? Making a sandwich will give me time to think it over."

Being able to recognize that sometimes we are the servants of our emotions, and cultivating the skill to have better control of our day, our mental state, and our reaction to feelings that come up, will make a difference between achieving great performance or mediocre outcomes. Because if we use the kettle as a crutch, before we know it, our day, together with our intentions and our goals, escapes us.

In his book, *Charged*, Brendon Burchard talks about intrinsic and extrinsic ways to manage emotional states, which I directly correlate to our choices around food. There are both constructive and destructive reactions to any event, depending on how we choose to respond. A false, or what I would consider a destructive extrinsic solution could be to reach for comfort food anytime there is a stressful or unpleasant event. The reason we do this is because our brain's circuitry is wired to avoid pain and choose what provides pleasure. During a stressful moment, we shift our focus to finding pleasure in our favorite snack rather than wholeheartedly and mindfully channeling our focus to what our brain perceives as a painful experience. I often explain to my clients that in our time, the buildings we work in, the cars we drive, and the places we shop are all very modern. However, certain aspects of our brains are primitive, such as the amygdala, known as the integrative center for emotions. The amount of stress an average human being experiences is drastically different and greater than what our ancestors experienced, yet the response to stress remains the same.

We are not hardwired to lean into pain, so we must cultivate the resiliency and the discipline to change our experience and reaction to perceived pain. By becoming the master of your emotions and choosing not to medicate your feelings with distractions in the form of food and other destructive behaviors, you create space for personal and professional growth. By addressing the psychology, you then influence your physiology by making better nutrition and lifestyle choices that lead to greater levels of performance. You achieve that by being strategic about your day—there is a time to fuel and nourish your mind and body, and there is a time to be fully engaged in your work, whatever that means to you.

Outlined below are the **top five steps** that you can take to optimize mental performance, increase energy, improve focus, decrease stress, and stop food cravings and other distractions from hijacking your precious time and waistline. These steps will not only help structure your day for maximum productivity but will also have tremendous positive impact on your health.

►**CHAPTER 9 EXERCISES:** 5 Steps to Less Stress, Slimmer Waistlines, and Increased Productivity:

1. Power sessions

I learned about power sessions at a time in my life when I was working on multiple projects at a time, running a business, seeing patients, being a mom, taking care of my family, and trying to find time to make it all happen every day. Identifying and minimizing distractions as well as staying on top of time management was of utmost importance if I wanted to continue being a supermom. This was when I discovered the Tony Robbins RPM, rapid planning method, and also decided that I needed a coach to teach me how to be the most efficient with my time and in my relationships. I contacted the Tony Robbins team, and after a very thorough interview process and multiple questionnaires, I got assigned my coach, Suzie.

For anyone looking to take the next step in life, be it personal or professional, it can be so helpful to have someone like Suzie on board to keep you accountable, on track, and most importantly, provide you with lightbulb moments.

I've had many lightbulb moments with Suzie. One of them was the concept of power sessions. During one of our conversations, I asked her "How in the heck do I get it all done, maintain my health and sanity, and grow my business?" One reason I loved working with Suzie was because she never skipped a beat and always had an answer to what seemed to be an insurmountable task.

She taught me the concept of power sessions, which are blocked time chunks during which you get an X amount of work done—no more, no less, and nothing else gets your attention. That means that if you sat down for a certain period of time and had a planned list of things that needed to get done in that time frame, you wouldn't get up and make coffee, grab a snack, send a quick message to a friend, oh, and make your grocery list so you wouldn't forget. Nope, because all those things are done before or after power sessions. Do you see how efficient you can be with power sessions and how it minimizes distractions?

Think of power sessions as exercise. You may not want to do it, but you kind of have to. It's best to do it daily for a certain amount of time. Once you're five minutes into it, it really isn't so bad—kind of like exercise. The best way to plan your daily power sessions is to take a look at your to-do list and choose a time during the day when you can allocate fifteen to fifty-five minutes to go through your list or at least part of it. During this time, your phone is silent, maybe your door is closed, and you've made it clear to anyone who may bother you that you're not available. Take care of the basics before starting the power session so that you can focus on the task at hand and not on how thirsty or hungry you are.

At the end of fifteen to fifty-five minutes (whatever time frame you choose), you stop and put your to-do list away. You've earned your break, and you can get back to your Instagram, dinner prep, friends, coffee, or whatever else was competing for your attention.

Power sessions are an excellent way to prevent distractions from taking another precious minute out of our day. After learning this, I've scheduled multiple power sessions during the day to help me stay in tune with what's important in the moment. Power sessions helped me get my perpetual snacking under control. If uncomfortable feelings surfaced as I was dealing with an unpleasant to-do, I worked through it rather than fueling my feelings with caffeine, social media, and my favorite chocolate, even if it was dark chocolate.

The great part about power sessions is that they keep you focused, you become efficient with your time, and when the session is up you move on with the rest of your day with a sense of accomplishment. Always a bonus.

2. Move Every Hour—Here's a Long Answer

I'm on a mission to get people moving more outside of the structured gym or fitness class. Although the gym or fitness class has tremendous value and benefit, the movement you do throughout the day contributes to increased metabolic rate and decreased muscle fatigue and helps regulate insulin and blood sugar levels. When your blood sugar is stable, you're less likely to make decisions you'll regret later.[5]

Even the most conditioned athletes are at risk for sitting too much. When I played tennis at the Bollettieri Academy, we had conditioning in the morning, tennis drills in the afternoon for four to six hours, followed by an evening workout Monday through Friday. Just when we thought we had earned our rest for the weekend, our trainers would rally us together to do a "recovery" workout. I remember the recovery workout as one of the hardest workouts of the week, because my body was sore, and the last thing I wanted to do was move. However, I found that I felt so much better within minutes of starting to move—just breaking a little bit of sweat stimulated endorphin production, and I went from feeling fatigued to feeling strong, energized, and motivated. This idea of moving even when you don't feel like it is a life-changing concept.

Exercise deficiency is something we must address not just on a daily basis but throughout the day. There's a cascade of biochemical reactions that happen when we opt for movement at least every hour. Here's a quick breakdown of the hormones involved and what they mean for your cravings, hunger, brain health, and waistline:

Ghrelin:

Ghrelin is a hormone that's produced in the stomach and sends a signal to the brain that you're hungry. Because exercise decreases overall ghrelin levels, it's one of the important factors to consider in weight loss and overall weight maintenance. Simply reducing caloric intake won't make a difference, but working out will. An interesting fact, however, and something you won't find in mainstream literature is that ghrelin levels decrease only short-term with exercise. Therefore, you need to be consistent with how often you exercise to achieve an ongoing effect.[6]

Leptin:

Leptin is another hormone to consider in appetite regulation, as it regulates energy balance and metabolism by inhibiting hunger. Leptin's actions are opposed by ghrelin, and both hormones effect the area of the brain called the hypothalamus in order to regulate appetite for optimal energy homeostasis. Makes sense, since ideally, we get most of our energy from food.

Leptin is released from fat cells, so the more body fat you have, the more likely you are to have leptin resistance at the brain level. Essentially, your brain stops responding to the increased levels of circulating leptin. Leptin sensitivity is best improved with training and diet strategies that lead to weight loss and weight maintenance. Research shows that exercise alone is not enough to significantly lower leptin. Actual weight loss needs to happen in order to see and feel the difference.[7]

Adiponectin:

This is one of the essential hormones involved in regulating blood glucose levels and fat breakdown. Adiponectin is secreted by fat cells, and its concentration is inversely related to the body mass index (BMI)—the higher the BMI, the lower the levels of the circulating hormone.[10] More research needs to be done to truly assess the relationship between exercise and adiponectin, but several studies have concluded that moderate-intense exercise does stimulate the production of adiponectin. This results in increased glucose uptake by cells, improved insulin sensitivity, and higher levels of fat breakdown for energy production,[17] all you need to live a healthy, productive, and energetic life.

Insulin & Glucagon:

I can't possibly talk about exercise and not mention these two vital hormones. Many people hear about insulin as it relates to diabetes, but few know about what glucagon does. The prefix "gluc" gives you a hint that it has to do with glucose. Exercise is by far one of the best ways to achieve a positive and synergistic relationship between insulin and glucagon.

Glucagon acts as the opposite of insulin. When the body registers blood glucose to be low, glucagon activates the breakdown of carbohydrates and fat into glucose. Exercise is one of the best ways to use up glucose and stimulate further carbohydrate and fat breakdown. When you incorporate physical activity throughout the day and consume more protein and fat in proportion to carbohydrates, you optimize fat breakdown for energy as orchestrated by glucagon.[18]

After exercise, glycogen gets replenished by glucose floating in the bloodstream, which is mediated by actions of insulin. Since insulin resistance is a big issue nowadays due to conventional diet, exercise deficiency, and lifestyle, incorporating movement throughout the day can help improve glucose uptake by cells and help regulate blood sugar.[17]

Epinephrine:

Life is about balance. Too little stress and we're sitting on the couch. Too much stress and we're paralyzed from fear. The truth is that we need a little bit of stress in life to keep our metabolism going. I'm talking about good stress, the kind that will give you just enough cortisol and epinephrine release without jeopardizing your health. Epinephrine is another hormone that increases in circulation when we exercise, making exercise a healthy stressor when done in moderation. This hormone is considered a fight or flight hormone like cortisol and is known to naturally suppress appetite and stimulate the release of fat for energy. It doesn't help convert fat into energy—that is a whole different process—but it does help make fat more available.[30]

So go ahead, peel yourself away from your desk, and gift yourself with a little bit of good stress that will help you see more clearly and perform better.

Growth hormone

This is the fountain of youth, as it's called. It also helps mobilize fat from fat cells and is produced during intense exercise and sleep! Here's another reason to get to bed early and improve sleep hygiene. My clients who have a hard time losing weight and experience food cravings during the day have an underlying long term sleep deficiency and stress that's left unchecked. Too little sleep and a lot of stress will make the stress hormones peak, while the growth hormone will tank—not a good scenario, but one that many people find themselves in.

Note that most studies cited show that moderate to intense exercise achieves the best results. When you opt to move throughout the day, add a little pep to your step to get the heart rate up. There are many short and long workouts available online to suit everyone's needs. Scroll through and watch a couple of videos to find some that you like and can do on a consistent basis. Consider hiring a trainer for a few sessions to make sure you have good form. A good trainer can also help you create a workout routine that you can do anywhere using your own body weight. When in doubt, simply find a set of stairs that you can run or walk to get your heart rate up, even if it's only for a few minutes.

One of the most important things that I recommend in this process is not to be hard on yourself but also not to let excuses get in the way of your success. Time is the number one excuse for people, and I am here to tell you that you've got ten minutes during the day when you can do a workout. It's amazing what you can do in ten minutes! In fact, you'll be amazed just how often you could do these ten-minute workout sessions during the day—upon rising, during lunch break, when you get home, or after the kids go to bed. The possibilities are vast and the results are undeniable.

3. No Food at Work Desk

Eating and working recruit completely opposing neurological pathways in the brain and body. We have a parasympathetic nervous system response when we eat, also known as the "rest and digest" response, which means no cognitively engaging tasks should be done at that time. When we are reading emails or trying to solve a complex problem, we are in a sympathetic nervous system mode, also called the "fight or flight" mode, and no major meal should be eaten at that time.

There is no such thing as multitasking, but there is the concept of doing multiple things mindfully. When you're eating and working at the same time, you're not doing either of the things mindfully, as your brain jumps from one task to the other and physiologically different pathways are involved.

Think of the power sessions mentioned earlier. Have a planned snack or meal during the day, and step away from your desk to have it. Your brain won't waste precious energy trying to focus on multiple tasks at a time, and your work performance will increase, as you'll focus on work rather than on your stomach.

I used to be a chronic snacker, so this concept resonates deeply. I also thought I had to eat my way through work and would have my lunch at the desk or have dinner while working on a project. In writing this book, I realized just how much room for improvement I had in my professional life and how snacking was hijacking my focus.

One of the things that helped me have my meals away from my desk was implementing power sessions, when I did not touch any food for an extended period of time while I worked through my to-do's. I'd have a proper meal before I got started, had my cup of coffee or tea on standby, and would breathe deeply when temptation would sneak in.

As I mentioned earlier, the concept of no food at the work desk has become policy in some workplaces like CBRE, a real estate services and investment company. Lisa Fulford-Roy, CBRE's managing director of workplace strategy, said, "The healthy desk policy is an internal CBRE policy implemented across our offices to encourage our staff to take a break from their desks, connect with colleagues and to promote healthier workstations."

The ultimate goal with policies like these is to lower stress and increase productivity, as employees are expected to take a break from their computers, relax, and hopefully share lunch with colleagues.[34]

One of my clients, a very successful CFO for a medical device start-up, took the time to structure his day around meetings, exercise, meditation, and meals. Although his schedule was as volatile as the nature of the start-up business, he was able to make time to have his lunch and snacks away from the desk to help re-focus and come back refreshed to his work. The result was decreased stress and increased capacity to problem solve.

You can achieve this too by simply following the **first three steps: create power sessions, move your body throughout the day, and plan your meals away from your workstation!**

4. Time chunking

Time chunking and power sessions are some of my favorite strategies for minimizing distractions and increasing daily productivity. I owe my knowledge about time chunking to Marie Forleo. I've mentioned Marie before, and that's because this woman is brilliant when it comes to creating a successful day. She also provides lots of resources to help her fans get the most out their time and money. Time chunking is one of the strategies I learned from her. It's similar to power sessions but not exactly the same. When you time chunk, every task from answering emails to exercise has its own time slot during the day. This is the time when you do that particular task and nothing else. As with power sessions, you do whatever it takes to keep your focus on the task at hand and not get distracted by people, phones, and food.

It's amazing how distractions surface when you time chunk. This is especially hard when you're at the office, since everyone is fighting to get your attention. Did you get my email? Could you help me with this problem? Oh, my gosh, can we please talk about what happened at the dinner party yesterday?

I used to feel bad for saying things like, "I'd love to chat, but I have limited time, and I'd love get this project done before the end of the day." People would guilt trip me too, as if I needed more guilt in my life! But becoming the owner of my time and placing high value on who and what gets my attention throughout the day has led to bigger outcomes than I imagined, so I am even more assertive in communicating boundaries around time.

The power of time chunking should not be underestimated. Too much time gets lost by checking emails every few minutes or catching up with distracted colleagues. Pay attention to the tasks that you schedule throughout the day but don't get to because A) deep down inside you're avoiding this task and would rather do something else, or B) you're not setting clear boundaries for time chunking to happen, so distractions take over.

As with power sessions, I recommend structuring your day into time chunks the night before or the morning of, depending on how much flexibility you need. Give yourself the lay of the land for what needs to happen, and allocate an approximate time for each task. Of course, this includes planning your meals around your work and life schedule so you're not caught off guard. How many of us have sat down to start on a project only to realize—wait a second, I'm hungry!

Include time chunking along with the other strategies for optimal health and productivity.

Before I move on to the last step, I'd like to share a sample of how I time chunk my day. Note that I do include all of the principles that I talk about: power sessions, movement, time chunking, and meals away from my desk.

5 a.m.—wake up, rise and shine!

5:30—warm up with yoga + bulletproof coffee

6-7:00 a.m.—breakfast for everyone

7:00-8 a.m.—workout session, get ready, out the door

9-10 a.m.—read, write, emails

11-1 p.m.—patients

1-2:30 p.m.—read, move, lunch, power session

2-5 p.m.—patients

5:30-7:30 p.m.—family time

7:30 p.m.-10 p.m.—prep for next day, meal prep, journal, yoga, anything else I didn't have time for

5. Rule of 52 and 17

Ideally, how long should your power sessions last? How much time should you spend working on a task?

Many of us find ourselves in a perpetual cycle of work with blurry lines where work starts and ends. But studies have shown that this is not how we achieve productivity, because the brain is like a muscle that over time gets tired with repeated use.

I am sure there is a time in your day when you hit a wall, then go for a walk around the block, and voila, the wall is no longer there when you come back. There is science behind this phenomenon. Here's a little blurb about productivity from The Atlantic: "The truth about productivity for the rest of us is that more hours doesn't mean better work. Rather, like a runner starting to flag after a few miles, our ability to perform tasks has diminishing returns over time. We need breaks strategically served between our work sessions."

Enter the 52 and 17 rule for productivity. DeskTime, an app that tracks employees' computer use, discovered that its most productive workers would spend 52 minutes working followed by 17 minutes of being away from their desk. People would spend that time talking to colleagues, exercising, and doing things outside of work.[45]

The article also mentioned a study that was done a while back by Cornell University's Ergonomics Research Laboratory, where workers received alerts to remind them to stand up and take a break. In comparison to workers who did not receive the alert, those who did were 13% more accurate in their work.

These are just two data points, but few will argue that taking intermittent breaks from work won't lead to increased performance. In your personal or professional life, it doesn't have to be this exact ratio of 52 minutes of work followed by 17 minutes of play. But taking a break at least every hour will lead to greater health and productivity outcomes.

What will you do next time you have 17 minutes of freedom? If you apply this concept on a daily basis, you will have multiple opportunities to eat, breathe, and move. Your break time is just as serious as your work time. Honor this time, and allow yourself the room to step away from the work station to take care of you.

From the concepts and strategies introduced in this section, time allocation is one of the key takeaway points for achieving optimal performance in personal and professional life. When you are strategic about your time, you find that you do have time to eat well, hydrate, sleep, work, and spend time with your loved ones. Simply spending a few minutes out of your day to plan breaks, power sessions, movement, or time chunks will lead to more fulfillment, decreased stress, and a happier life. I think we all want that.

Conclusion

There is a story behind every craving. Having a total mind-body approach rather than just looking at one possible reason is usually the answer. Cravings are a way that our body can communicate with us. They're a body's way of saying, "Hey, pay attention!" When we do pay attention, when we ask the right questions, and when we know where to go to find the answers, we can reap the benefits of great health and minimize unnecessary suffering. Knowledge is power, and you now have the knowledge to go system by system to uncover weaknesses and use the tools and resources provided in every chapter to patch any holes to start feeling optimal.

I am a true believer – and I have heard this from other colleagues and my professors – that 80 percent of the time, patients know what's wrong, and the other 20 percent is for the healthcare provider to figure out. Taking the time to understand your personal story is the first step in the journey to better health. In taking time to reflect, you'll see the hidden interconnections between nutrition, mood, gut health, hormones, brain health, and, of course, the foods you're craving.

Whatever your story and your journey has been, no matter how simple or intricate, know that there is always something you can do and that you can always dig deeper for answers. You might be thinking, "I've seen a dozen different doctors, and no one seems to find the answer." Maybe you have not found the right doctor or a team that understands how the body is meant to function and knows the resources to help you get to the optimal state. Maybe you haven't given your health provider enough time to help you resolve whatever challenge you're facing. Frequently, people are sick for years but have the expectation that they should be healed within days or weeks. I've seen cases in which a person will go from one provider to the next, expecting to be cured, when they have not given the provider a chance to look into all the layers that are interconnected. Be patient with yourself as you make the change to your nutrition, fitness, and lifestyle and as you address the more complex issues regarding hormone health, gut health, brain health, and nutrient imbalances.

What we know about the human body and all the systems, physical and non-physical, continues to evolve, and as new evidence, research, and knowledge surfaces, there are some things that always remain true. One of these truths is that your body and the cells that comprise it are always trying to get back to a state of health or equilibrium in the process called homeostasis. Listening to your body's signs as it tries to find equilibrium is one of the greatest gifts you can give to yourself. I consider food cravings to be one of the major signs. Each chapter has demonstrated all the possible ways that you can get back to equilibrium.

Each and every one of us has the gifts or talents that we inherently want and need to share with the world. I firmly stand by my belief that in order to serve our purpose in life, we need to strive to be a better version of ourselves each and every day. You are more equipped to face any challenge that comes your way when you have a healthy mind and body, free from any limitations and cravings.

The *14-Day Crave Reset*™ *Sugar Cleanse*

Please note that the 14-Day Crave Reset™ *Sugar Cleanse is not intended for the treatment or prevention of disease, nor is it a replacement for seeking medical treatment or professional nutrition advice. Do not start any nutrition or physical activity program without first consulting your physician.*

Our skin, liver, lungs, gut, and kidneys work 24/7 to filter, cleanse, and provide the optimal environment for our bodies to thrive. These vital organs are constantly taxed by our decision to exercise or not, the environment we live in, and the food that we put in our bodies, to mention just a few.

Most people sign up for a cleanse or a detox challenge and after that's done, resort to old habits until the next cleanse. Billions of cells make up the connective tissue and organs in our body, and these cells go through their own life cycle. Some have a shorter life span than others, but all of them only last for a certain period of time before being replaced.

Every day is an opportunity to improve your physiology, metabolism, and internal and external environment. Because the life of any given cell is not permanent, you have an opportunity to start new daily. When you commit to supporting the body in detoxing or eliminating toxins daily, you provide the perfect environment for optimal energy production, fat breakdown, nutrient absorption, mental clarity, better sleep, and the list goes on.

THE GOALS:

The goal over the next fourteen days is multifold: 1) cleanse your palette, 2) clear your mind & body, 3) reset your palette, 4) curb your cravings, and 5) achieve freedom from sugar using the Crave Reset™ dietary guidelines and nutritional support. The guidelines as well as the supplements are an effective way to detox and can be turned into a 7-day cleanse throughout the year whenever you need a quick reset.

Anytime an addictive substance, such as sugar, is taken out completely, it creates an initial stress in the human body on a hormonal and also neurotransmitter level. Nobody feels good for the first few days, and sometimes weeks, after giving up sugar. That's because of the effect sugar has on the feel-good neurotransmitters serotonin and dopamine. Balancing blood sugar and maintaining optimal serotonin and dopamine balance with the right foods and nutritional support will be the key to the 14-day sugar-free success.

If you recall from earlier chapters, carbohydrates normally make serotonin levels spike, which is why we always come back for more. Protein and fat do not have that same effect. That is why the basic Crave Reset™ dietary guidelines include the following. (Remember, it's only fourteen days!)

NO STARCHY VEGETABLES:

This means no yams, sweet potatoes, potatoes, butternut squash, corn, and other starchy vegetables high in sugar, such as beets and carrots. You can also have limited varieties of legumes including beans and lentils, which are listed in food choices below. Focus on the abundance of veggies that you can have, such as leafy greens like kale and collard greens, beet greens, and cruciferous vegetables like broccoli, brussels sprouts, and cabbage, all of which are low in sugar and support the liver's detox pathways.

LEAN & CLEAN PROTEIN:

Eat an organic protein of choice for lunch to balance blood sugar. If you are vegan/vegetarian, limit legumes, such as lentils and beans, to one serving per day. Do this even if you do not have dietary restrictions. This cleanse is meant to be sustainable!

GET PLENTY OF HEALTHY FAT:

Fat makes up every cellular membrane in our bodies. Our brain relies on omega-3 fats to build new cells and function optimally. Get plenty of healthy fats from produce like avocado, eggs, nuts, seeds, and fish to help balance mood, hormones, and neurotransmitter production.

NO PROCESSED SUGAR OR SWEETENERS:

Sugar is sneaky and makes its way in multiple forms into everything. Protein bars, granola bars, sports drinks and others contain sweeteners like maltodextrin, brown rice syrup, and coconut palm sugar. You can have limited amounts of honey, maple syrup, or stevia.

ENJOY LOW SUGAR FRUIT:

Have one to two servings of fruit, limited to berries, pears, and apples. Other fruits have higher sugar content and are best avoided during the cleanse. Dried fruit is concentrated with sugar and should be avoided.

START AND END YOUR DAY WITH PROTEIN:

For the next thirty days, start your morning with a protein shake and choose two days a week when you can have a protein shake for both breakfast and dinner.

CRAVE RESET™ SIMPLE SCHEDULE & RECIPES

The Crave Reset™ protocol is designed to minimize cravings naturally by promoting a healthy stress response and balancing neurotransmitters. In this section, you will find recipes for smoothies, snacks, and the major meals of the day.

Over fourteen days, breakfast and dinner will be smoothies made with organic ingredients and a protein powder of choice. If you don't want to do smoothies, you can just do the protein powder by itself. Having two meal replacements will not only give your digestion a break but will further facilitate elimination of metabolic waste, as the body will clear excess fat deposits.

How do you choose the best protein powder?

It's very important that you add a protein powder that does not have any sugar or other additives. The more minimal the better. Consider experimenting with some of the smoothies listed below, and make your own versions as you go. If you want to have your smoothies for breakfast and lunch instead of breakfast and dinner, you can! It's about what is most convenient given your schedule and preferences.

There are more recipes listed at the end of the book, so be sure to check those out if you need more inspiration or would like to try something new!

SCHEDULE:

Breakfast:
Meal replacement smoothie with protein of choice. See recipes below.

Lunch:
Choose items from the suggested food choices and refer to meal and snack suggestions on the next pages.

Dinner:
Meal replacement smoothie with protein of choice. See recipes below.

Snacks:
This is not meant to be calorie restrictive. Snacking is allowed. Refer to meal and snack suggestions on the next pages.

SUGGESTED FOOD AND SNACK CHOICES:

Protein:
Organic, Hormone Free

Consider cooking with the following protein choices during the 14-day cleanse. I normally would not recommend soy products, however, if you are vegan or vegetarian, I suggest including more fermented soy products like tempeh over tofu for sources of protein. Packaged vegan/vegetarian products like tofurky can be full of soy and wheat, so opting for whole food items for at least the 14-day cleanse can be highly beneficial.

Bison
Chicken

Halibut or Cod

Chicken

Turkey

Salmon

Lamb

Chicken and/or duck eggs

Sardines or other cold water fish

Vegetables:
Low starch, Low sugar, Organic

The point of the cleanse is to reduce our dependency on processed and sugary foods. Although most vegetables are okay, some that are not have a way of sneaking into our diet and impact our blood sugar and insulin levels in a negative way. Take the sweet potato or yam, for example. (I am just as guilty of overindulging in it.) Not all root vegetables and squash are created equal. Some naturally contain more starch and sugar than others – it's just part of being a plant. The list below provides vegetable choices that tend to be lower in starch and therefore won't have as negative an impact on your blood sugar as others do. Of course, a sweet potato is better than a donut, but what we're doing here is taking out the foods that we normally incline toward, which is where we usually run into trouble. Enjoy the following in abundance:

Arugula

Spinach

Broccoli'

Cucumber

Beet greens

Swiss chard

Cauliflower

Cabbage

Collard greens

Bok choy

Mushrooms

Zucchini

Chard

Brussels sprouts

Celery'

Avocado

Summer squash

Onions

Kale

Grains:

Gluten free

Unless you are sensitive or allergic to certain grains, have a health condition that grains make worse, or overconsume them on a regular basis, you can include grains in moderation. Grains that are flawed are overly processed, refined, or genetically modified grains—think typical wheat or white bread, white rice, and pasta. Gluten free grains, such as those listed below, are packed with protein and healthy carbohydrates. Including a serving a day, depending on the grain, is completely allowed on the 14-day cleanse. You may consider excluding them to test for food sensitivities, but that is optional. Have a serving of the following:

Amaranth

Brown or wild rice

Millet

Quinoa

Buckwheat

Teff

Nuts and Seeds:
Unsalted, raw

Nuts and seeds make for a great snack and are packed with important fats, such as omega-3's. Sprinkle these over salads or roasted vegetables, or have a handful when you need something quick and healthy. Roasted nuts sold in stores tend to be more prone to having mold contamination, so be sure to purchase raw whenever possible. If you want to roast the nuts or seeds yourself, go for it! Just remember that the process of roasting can destroy some of the important fats. It's easy to overindulge in nuts and seeds—don't find yourself just eating aimlessly out of the pack. Enjoy the following in moderation:

Almonds

Hazelnuts

Chia seeds

Pecans

Cashews

Pumpkin seeds

Pistachios

Pine nuts

Sunflower seeds

Walnuts

Flax seeds

Legumes:
Non-canned Beans and Lentils

Use in moderation and sparingly, similar to the use of grains, meaning they should not be your primary fuel sources, as they are higher in carbohydrates and starch than other fuel sources already mentioned. Because legumes contain phytic acid, which can prevent the binding of key nutrients like zinc, iron, and Vitamin A, soak them twelve to twenty-four hours prior to cooking to help remove phytic acid and avoid nutritional deficiencies. Here's the list of allowed legumes. Have a serving a day if they are currently part of your meal plan.

Black-eyed peas

Lima beans

Green peas

Lentils

Edamame

Mung beans

Fruit:

No Tropical or Citrus Fruits

Fruit is exceptionally good for us but can also be super easy to overeat. Some fruit is better than others when it comes to sugar content and nutrient density. Although tropical fruits and citrus fruits have certain benefits, one of the reasons they are excluded for the next fourteen days is because they tend to have a higher amount of sugar—and we are trying to kick the sugar habit! I recommend limiting fruit to one or two servings a day. Think of one cup of berries or one medium size apple as a serving. When you're craving something sweet have a piece of fruit!

Apples

Pears

Blueberries

Strawberries

Raspberries

Blackberries

Condiments:

Dressings, Sauces

Dressings, sauces, and toppings are where people start running into trouble. There are many great and simple recipes for dressings that contain flavorful ingredients. Most dressings contain oils like canola or safflower, which are pro-inflammatory. Pairing herbs like cilantro, dill, and thyme with good-for-you vinegars like unfiltered apple cider vinegar and healthy oils like extra virgin oil will not only provide excellent flavor but also great health benefits.

Apple cider vinegar

Avocado oil

Fresh herbs and spices

Extra virgin olive oil

Butter or ghee

Coconut oil

Sweeteners:

No Artificial Sweeteners

This is the sections that gets everyone's attention. The 14-day cleanse is meant to be a springboard for your new way of eating and living. It's not meant to be limiting, so naturally sweet produce like raw honey and maple syrup are allowed, all in moderation, of course. I've led many cleanses and nutrition programs that considered these to be banned substances during a sugar cleanse, but what I have found, and what clients have reported back, is that they were more likely to binge or go back to old eating habits when following a very strict sugar elimination. Your palette will recalibrate by simply removing the processed sugar, such as cane sugar, brown rice syrup, and other sweeteners like maltodextrin and tapioca syrup. And, yes, stevia is allowed. Allow yourself one to three teaspoons of the following:

Honey

Maple syrup

Snacks:

Using Whole Foods

While on the cleanse, consider including healthy, whole foods snacks with cleanse-friendly ingredients like the ones listed in this section. You can include a snack midmorning and/or midday to help keep your blood sugar balanced. This will not only prevent overindulging during major meals but will also improve your mood, concentration, and focus, all while keeping your insulin and blood sugar at a happy balance. Prepping becomes key, and it can be helpful to plan your snacks the night before so you can grab and go:

Cucumber slices with hummus and avocado

Brown rice cakes with nut butter and apple

Nut milk yogurt with berries and seeds

Homemade trail mix (recipe in the back)

Hard-boiled egg with avocado

Fresh fruit and nuts

Celery and zucchini sticks or roasted veggies with hummus

1 ounce of meat like chicken or turkey (non-deli)

Paleo granola (see recipe in the back)

Homemade protein bars (see recipes in the back)

Recipes for the Cleanse

BREAKFAST AND DINNER SMOOTHIE RECIPES:

I frequently ask, "How do you smoothie?" Smoothies are such a great way to jump-start your day, to use as a snack, or in this case, to have as a meal replacement. You can easily double the recipe and store the rest in the refrigerator at work or home. Smoothies are also a great way to sneak in veggies that you normally don't like. Think of a vegetable that you know you could use more of, and try it in a smoothie. Of course, not all vegetables will go well, but most vegetables that have a relatively neutral flavor like spinach and kale work great!

Berry Extravaganza
Servings: 1

1/2 cup blueberries, fresh or frozen

1/2 cup strawberries, fresh or frozen

1 Tbsp almond butter

1 scoop protein powder

1 cup unsweetened almond milk or coconut milk

Water as needed

Combine all ingredients in a blender and blend until desired consistency, about 30 seconds. If you don't want to use almond butter, you can soak a couple of tablespoons of nuts the night before and add them to the smoothie in the morning.

Kale Zinger

Servings: 1

1/2 cup blackberries, fresh or frozen

1/2 cup blueberries, fresh or frozen

Handful of spinach or kale

1 cup unsweetened almond milk or coconut milk

1/2 tsp grated ginger

1 scoop protein powder

Water as needed

Place all ingredients in a blender and combine until desired consistency is reached, about 30 seconds. Ginger is great at giving smoothies a little heat and pairs well with the greens and berries. If you have a greens powder that you like, you can include it here as well.

Green Fuel

Servings: 1

1/2 green apple

1/2 pear

Handful of kale

1/4 avocado

2 Tbsp hemp seeds

1 scoop protein powder

1 tsp spirulina powder

1 1/2 cups of water

Additional water as needed

Chop the apple and pear. Place all ingredients in a blender and combine for 1 minute. The avocado will make this smoothie relatively thick, so add water to thin it out as needed. You can also place the apple and pear in the freezer the night before to make the smoothie more refreshing. In the summertime, I blend most of my smoothies with frozen fruits, but during the cooler months, I use fresh fruit.

LUNCH/DINNER RECIPES:

Roasted Veggies and Salmon with a Creamy Apple Cider Vinegar Vinaigrette

Servings: 4

This is an excellent recipe that can be used for lunch, dinner, and leftovers! If you don't have salmon, substitute another protein source. The dressing also makes a great marinade for tofu for anyone looking for a vegan or vegetarian option. You can bake the tofu like the veggies; just turn once a while to ensure that it bakes evenly.

4 cups quartered brussels sprouts

3 cups broccoli cut into bite size pieces

4 fillets of grilled or baked salmon, preferably not previously frozen, and not farmed

2 tsp cumin

2 tsp ginger

2 tsp turmeric

4 Tbsp olive oil

For the dressing:

1/3 cup apple cider vinegar, raw

2 Tbsp honey, raw

1 clove garlic, finely minced

1 Tbsp Dijon mustard

Pinch of kosher or sea salt

1/4 tsp black pepper

2/3 cup extra-virgin olive oil

1/4 cup pumpkin seeds

Heat oven to 425°F. Toss brussels sprouts and broccoli in olive oil, cumin, turmeric, and ginger. Bake for 35-40 minutes until the veggies are done and slightly browned. While the brussels sprouts are baking, preheat the grill to medium heat and prepare salmon by coating the fillets with a little olive oil and sea salt. Grill for about five minutes on each side to desired doneness—more time for well-done and less time for medium. You can also bake the salmon with the brussels sprouts at 425°F for 15-20 min. When everything is cooked, combine all the dressing ingredients in a blender. Drizzle the veggies and salmon with the dressing and serve.

Earthy Lentil Salad with Shiitake Mushrooms and Avocado

This is another great dish to serve hot or cold and makes for a great stand-alone meal or a side dish. Add more greens as necessary and other vegetables and spices like curry that you may like. As with eggs and dairy, only consume lentils if you do not experience any digestive disturbance.

1/2 cup French Green Lentils

2 cups vegetable stock or water

4 cups shiitake mushrooms

2 tsp olive oil

1/2 shallot finely chopped

2 cloves of garlic finely chopped

1/4 tsp chili flakes or more to taste

1 1/2 Tbsp lemon juice

3 tsp extra virgin olive oil

sea salt and pepper to taste

2 Tbsp flat leaf parsley roughly chopped

1/2 cup kale, stems removed

Place the lentils and vegetable stock in a saucepan and bring to a boil Lower the heat and simmer for 25 minutes or until the lentils are tender. While the lentils are cooking, place a large frying pan over medium-high heat. Heat the oil, then add the shallot, garlic, chili flakes, and mushrooms. Cook until the mushrooms are tender. Toss the lentils and mushroom mixture with the lemon juice and kale. Season to taste and add the parsley for extra flavor!

Tangy Coleslaw with Roasted Chicken:
Servings: 4

This is a great alternative to traditional coleslaw. Cruciferous vegetables like cabbage are great for supporting good bacteria in our digestive tract, and they also support the liver. If you don't have access to avocado oil mayonnaise, you can use the Apple Cider Vinaigrette dressing instead. If a rotisserie chicken is all you have time for, go for it!

For the coleslaw:

1.5 cup shredded green cabbage

1.5 cup shredded purple cabbage

1 cup shredded apple

1/4 cup of Avocado Oil Mayonnaise or see recipe above for Apple
     Cider Vinaigrette

2 Tbsp apple cider vinegar (skip if using the vinaigrette)

1 Tbsp honey or maple syrup

1/4 cup chopped cilantro

1/4 cup sunflower seeds

Sea salt to taste

For the roasted chicken:

1/2 cup freshly squeezed lime juice

2 cloves of garlic finely chopped

4 Tbsp honey

2 Tbsp soy sauce

2 Tbsp olive oil

7 or 8 chicken thighs

1/2 tsp sea salt

green onions, chopped

Heat oven to 425°F. In a small bowl, combine lime juice, honey, garlic, olive oil, and soy sauce to make a marinade. Rub the chicken thighs with sea salt. Pour the marinade into a glass baking dish, add chicken thighs, and make sure to cover thoroughly. For more flavor, you can let the thighs marinate overnight. Bake for 25-30 minutes until the chicken is done.

While the chicken is baking, in a salad bowl mix the cabbage and carrots with the apple cider vinegar or a couple tablespoons of the vinaigrette. To improve digestibility of the vegetables, using your hands, massage the cabbage and carrots. Add the avocado oil mayonnaise, maple syrup or honey, cilantro, and sunflower seeds. Mix thoroughly and set aside.

When the chicken is done, let it cool for a few minutes, garnish with chopped green onions. Plate the coleslaw and chicken thighs, and savor this healthy wonder!

Hearty Quinoa & Tahini Bowl

Servings: 2 big bowls

This is a great meal that you can prep ahead of time. Cook the quinoa the night before, chop the veggies over the weekend, make the dressing ahead of time, and store in the fridge to be used for salads and bowls like these. A great, fast dinner for nights when you want something good, nourishing, and easy to make. Toss it up with avocado and even some other protein like tempeh, chicken, or salmon. The bowl is like a canvas; use what you got!

15 oz can chickpeas, drained, rinsed, paper towel dried

1 cup uncooked quinoa

1 large cucumber, peeled and julienned

2 cups purple cabbage

2 handfuls arugula

1/4 cup tahini

1/4 cup olive oil

half of lemon juice

Sliced avocado

Sea salt to taste

Spices like chili powder, garlic, cayenne to taste

1/2 cup chopped cilantro

2 Tbsp sunflower seeds

Preheat oven to 400°F and line two large baking sheets with parchment paper.

Transfer chickpeas to the baking sheet and drizzle with 1/2 teaspoon of olive oil, lightly coating them. Sprinkle with fine grain sea salt and your spices of choice. Toss to combine and place in the oven for 15 minutes. Gently roll around the chickpeas and place back in the oven for another 15 minutes. When the chickpeas are golden, they are ready to come out. Cool for 5 minutes.

To make the dressing, whisk together or blend the tahini, olive oil, and lemon juice. To assemble each bowl, add quinoa to the bottom of the bowl, then add arugula, cabbage, cucumber, chickpeas, and cilantro, coat with couple of tablespoons of the dressing, then top with avocado and sunflower seeds. Bon appetit!

Savory Chicken Curry in Lettuce Wraps

Servings: 6

Why are lettuce wraps so good? They make a great alternative to the typical sandwich! I frequently use lettuce wraps as carriers instead of bread, wraps, or chips. You can use basic iceberg lettuce, butter lettuce, kale, or collard greens, just remove the stalks. If you're looking to make to-go lettuce wraps, you can use a toothpick to keep the leaves from opening and keep it all together while it's in a container. I've taken lettuce wraps on hikes and to meetings, and they've accompanied me on many road trips!

4 chicken thighs

1 lemon, quartered

1/2 bunch cilantro leaves

Sea salt and freshly ground black pepper

1/4 cup avocado oil mayonnaise

1 tsp curry powder

1 tsp honey

1 tsp freshly squeezed lime or lemon juice

3 scallions, thinly sliced

2 stalks celery, thinly sliced

3/4 cup halved seedless red grapes

Butter lettuce leaves, for serving

Put the chicken thighs, lemon, cilantro leaves and stems into a saucepan. Fill with water to cover the chicken, and season with salt and pepper. Bring to a boil over medium heat, then reduce to simmer. Cook until the chicken is tender and is falling apart, about 40 minutes. Remove the chicken from the saucepan and allow to cool.

In a bowl, mix the avocado oil mayonnaise, curry, honey, and lemon or lime juice. Stir in the scallions, celery, and grapes until combined. Add the chicken meat and toss to combine. Season with salt and pepper and serve heaping portions of the salad in butter lettuce leaves.

Roasted Cod with Ginger Bok Choy

Servings: 2

Need help finding a simple teriyaki sauce alternative? This recipe features a similar sweetness and saltiness to classical teriyaki sauce minus all the gunk like tons of sugar, sodium, soy, and flavorings. You don't have to part with your favorite foods; you simply need to change the ingredients to achieve the same result but won't have you crashing and craving for more! If you don't have access to cod, substitute another fish or protein source. This also makes a great vegetarian dish if you want to substitute an array of vegetables for cod and turn this into a spectacular side dish.

2 cod fillets

1/3 cup coconut aminos, a soy sauce alternative

2 Tbsp maple syrup

2 Tbsp sesame oil

2 cloves garlic, crushed

2 Tbsp extra virgin olive oil

1 Tbsp grated ginger

1 Tbsp apple cider vinegar

6 oz baby bok choy

2 scallions chopped

In a glass baking dish, combine maple syrup, coconut aminos, sesame oil, and crushed garlic. Add cod fillets and coat in sauce. Allow to marinate for 30 minutes or up to 2 hours. Transfer fish to a foil-lined baking sheet. Roast at 475°F until cooked through and slightly browned, about 10 minutes.

Meanwhile, heat olive oil in a large skillet over medium heat; add ginger and cook for about 1 minute. Add bok choy and apple cider vinegar. Cook, stirring occasionally for 3-4 minutes until the greens are wilted and stalks are tender but crisp. Divide bok choy and cod between two plates and sprinkle with scallions.

Zucchini Noodles (Zoodles) with Chicken

Servings: 2

Zucchini is such a versatile vegetable. It's like a canvas for flavor. Zucchini noodles have become popular these days, and there are many ways you can prepare them. This is one of many. If you don't have access to a spiralizer or a store near you does not already have prepared zucchini noodles, feel free to chop them up, cook for a few minutes on a skillet, and use with the rest of the recipe. You can make this a dairy free recipe by substituting your favorite dairy alternative for the plain Greek yogurt.

1/4 cup plain Greek yogurt

3 Tbsp fresh lemon juice, plus additional for drizzling

2 tsp honey

3/4 tsp chia Seeds

1 tsp olive oil, plus additional for drizzling

3/4 tsp garlic minced

Salt and pepper to taste

8 oz Chicken breast

2 large zucchinis or 3 medium

1/3 cup reduced-fat feta cheese or goat cheese

Spiralizer or mandolin (Some stores sell spiralized zucchini noodles.)

In a medium bowl, whisk together the yogurt, lemon juice, honey, chia seeds, olive oil, garlic, and a pinch of salt and pepper. Place the chicken into the bowl and cover it with the mixture. Cover and refrigerate for at least 2 hours, so that the chicken has a chance to absorb the flavors.

Heat oven to 350°F, and place chicken along with the marinade into a baking dish.

Bake until chicken is done, about 25 minutes, and allow to cool for 5 minutes. Reserve the juices and marinade to make a sauce.

While the chicken is cooking, spiralize the zucchini noodles using the 3mm blade of the spiralizer or mandolin. You can skip this if you were able to get store-bought zoodles. Place the noodles into a strainer and set onto a medium bowl to collect water. Lightly sprinkle the zucchini noodles with salt and let strain for 30 minutes to release the water, stirring occasionally.

Squeeze out as much remaining liquid from the zucchini noodles as you can and place into a bowl. Drizzle with a little bit of olive oil and lime juice. Toss to evenly coat and divide between two plates.

Whisk the juice and marinade in a small bowl, adding any additional seasoning to taste. Place the chicken on top of the zucchini noodles and divide the sauce over the top of each plate. Sprinkle with feta or goat cheese, and savor the joy of this meal!

Crave Reset™ Recipe Collection

Tame the Sweet, Salty, Crunchy, and Everything in Between

In this section, you'll find recipes that are quick, easy to make, and most importantly, satisfying. These are great recipes to add to your daily meal plans, as they are balanced in protein, carbohydrates, and plenty of healthy fats—everything you need to keep your blood sugar stable. They do not require any fancy ingredients, and are totally versatile. If you don't like any one of the ingredients, feel free to change them. If you are doing the 14-day sugar cleanse mentioned earlier, remember to use low starch vegetables and avoid starchy vegetables for best results.

The nuts and fats used in these recipes are anti-inflammatory when consumed on a regular basis, as are the spices like ginger and turmeric. Spices like cinnamon are great for breakfast as they help to regulate blood sugar and can help keep you in equilibrium throughout the day.

Make these recipes ahead of time, such as with meal prep on weekends, to save time during the week. You can also double the recipes to have extra for leftovers, or use them to make smaller meals. If you have a tendency to overindulge at mealtime and you eat large meals, spacing your meals out and having four to five smaller meals during the day may be helpful. You will be less likely to overindulge, and you'll keep your caloric intake at bay.

I frequently post my favorite meals and snacks online, so follow me on Instagram and Facebook for inspiration and motivation! I also have a prolific Pinterest board that is filled with great recipes for all occasions. My intention is to provide as many tips and tools as I can to help you fine tune your palette and daily nutrition.

One thing I recommend to help my clients get variety is to get friends on board and exchange recipe and meal ideas. That way, you don't get bored with recipes, you can stock your freezer, and you have the added benefit of making it a social event.

To your health, enjoy!

MIGHTY BREAKFAST RECIPES

You'll notice is that I did not include eggs in my morning recipes. Eggs are a great source of protein and fat, and if you're not sensitive to them and don't have allergies, feel free to include them. Because I do a lot of food elimination in my practice, I know that eggs end up being one of the items that disappears from the menu. Note that smoothies are not listed here but are mentioned earlier and can absolutely be your breakfast. Some of these recipes make for great snacks, too, so experiment and find what works best for you!

Coconut Cacao Granola Grain Free

Servings: 16

This is a great recipe to use any time of day, for breakfast or snack. Pair it with fresh fruit or nut milk, toss with non-dairy yogurt, or have it as is! It makes for a great dessert and is easy to bring with you as a snack for a pre- and post-workout treat.

1 1/2 cups coconut flakes

1/2 cup almond slivers

1/4 cup pumpkin seeds

1/4 cup ground chia seeds

1/2 tsp vanilla

1/2 tsp cinnamon

1/2 tsp sea salt

5 medjool dates chopped

1/4 cup goji berries

3 Tbsp coconut oil

1/4 cup maple syrup or honey

1/4 cup raw cacao nibs

Preheat oven to 325°F, and line a baking sheet with parchment paper. Combine 1 cup of coconut, almonds, pumpkin seeds, sunflower seeds, ground chia seeds, goji berries, spices, and salt in a large mixing bowl. Add the pitted and chopped dates to the mixture and distribute thoroughly. Melt the coconut oil and pour the liquid ingredients, including maple syrup or honey, into the dry mixture. Stir to evenly coat, and transfer the mixture to the baking sheet. Bake for 30 minutes, stirring once in a while. Remove and let the granola cool. Stir in the remaining 1/2 cup of coconut flakes and cacao nibs, and store in an airtight container in the refrigerator to maintain freshness.

Berry Protein Smoothie Bowl

Servings: 2

Smoothie bowls can be a great alternative to typical breakfast recipes. They are light and refreshing and are packed with nutrients. This makes for a great meal during warm months and is even good as a light dinner. You can also use this recipe when following the 14-day cleanse mentioned earlier.

1 frozen Acai berry packet

1 cup frozen strawberries

Handful of spinach or kale

1 date

1 banana

2 tsp spirulina powder

1.5 scoops vanilla protein powder

Coconut milk or almond milk, enough to blend

Optional toppings like granola, seeds, berries

Blend all ingredients to a consistency that's thicker than a smoothie. Split the mixture between two bowls and top with optional toppings. Enjoy before it melts, but it's good either way!

Overnight Super Quinoa

Servings: 2

This is a perfect recipe that requires little prep work and is great for those mornings when you need something ready to go. Chia seeds and quinoa make a perfect combination and are packed with healthy fats, protein, and carbohydrates—everything you need to start your day right!

1 cup coconut milk

1/2 cooked quinoa

1/2 cup almond meal

4 Tbsp chia seeds, whole or ground

2 Tbsp maple syrup

1 scoop vanilla pea protein

1/4 tsp vanilla extract

Dash of sea salt

1 cup berries

Chopped almonds

Divide all ingredients except berries and chopped almonds between two jars, and stir until well combined. Place in the refrigerator and let sit overnight. Remove and top with berries and chopped almonds.

Cauliflower Morning Hash

Servings: 2

This is a great egg alternative recipe for breakfast, brunch, or any time for that matter. You can double the recipe and have leftovers the next day to save cooking and prep time. You can also take leftovers with you to have for lunch. Having versatile recipes like this one makes it easy to cook and eat well. Some stores sell already minced cauliflower that resembles rice, but you can also make it yourself by simply taking cauliflower florets and putting them through a food processor until they are chopped into rice size pieces.

1 avocado

1 lime

1/4 tsp garlic powder

Sea salt and pepper to taste

2 Tbsp cilantro chopped

2 chicken sausages, cooked, skin removed

2 Tbsp extra virgin olive oil

1 1/2 cups cauliflower rice

1 cup crimini mushrooms, sliced

2 cups spinach

1 green onion chopped

Optional salsa

In a small bowl, combine avocado, lime juice, garlic powder, salt, pepper, and chopped cilantro. Mash with a fork until all ingredients are combined and there are few or no chunks of avocado. Warm a medium sized skillet to medium temperature and add the olive oil. Toss in the mushrooms and cauliflower rice and cook until both are nearly done. Cut the cooked chicken sausage into quarter size circles and with the spinach, add to the skillet. Reduce heat to low-medium, and season with more garlic powder, sea salt, and pepper to taste. Cook until spinach is barely wilted, about 1 minute. Remove from heat, divide the cooked goodness between two bowls, and top with green onion. Serve it with the avocado mix.

Pump It Up Buckwheat Pancakes
Serves: 6 pancakes, 2 servings

This is one of my favorite recipes to make on the weekends. These pancakes are great on their own as a pre-workout meal or paired with other breakfast fixings if you're not in a hurry to start your weekend. You can make a few extra to take with you if you're going for a hike or skiing, or simply save some for the next day—they are great even when reheated. This is also kids' top pick and a great alternative to old fashioned pancakes.

1/2 cup buckwheat flour

1 Tbsp rice or almond flour

1 Tbsp arrowroot flour

20 g vanilla or plain pea protein powder

1/2 tsp baking powder

Dash of cinnamon

1/2 tsp vanilla extract

6 drops liquid stevia, plain or vanilla

Coconut oil or butter for cooking

Optional frozen blueberries

Heat a medium size, non-stick skillet, and melt enough coconut oil to lightly line the surface. Blend all the ingredients and add frozen blueberries last to combine. Scoop about 1/4 cup of batter per pancake and add to the skillet. Cook for 2-3 minutes per side on medium heat and flip carefully.

Allow pancakes to cool, and serve as is or add fresh berries. Drizzle lightly with maple syrup.

AFTERNOON CRASH AVERTED LUNCH RECIPES:

There are many reasons why someone can experience an afternoon crash. I've shared a lot of information for the different factors that can impact blood sugar. Diet is, of course, one of the first things to look at, and what you have (or don't have) for lunch can impact how you feel after lunch—what a concept! These recipes can be interchanged with dinner recipes and vice versa. The challenge everyone faces is work lunch meetings. My recommendation in this regard is to keep it simple—salad, protein, and a healthy carb—the cleanse basics. Most restaurants are accommodating, and you can more often than not choose a healthy option. Limit dressings and sauces to oils and vinegars, or vinaigrette when you can.

Kalelideiscope Salad Crunch
Servings: 4

Oh, the colors! Green, red, and blue from veggies and fruits combined! This is definitely an example of eating your rainbow. One reason I love making salads with kale is because kale tastes great the next day and doesn't get soggy like other greens. You can even give it some heat and steam kale before making the salad if eating it raw upsets your stomach. If you're not a fan of the nuts, throw in pumpkin or sunflower seeds. You can also substitute other berries for the blueberries and a pear for the apple—many different variations!

1 large apple, cut into small squares

1 avocado, cut into bite size pieces

1/4 cup fresh blueberries

1 large bunch kale, stems removed, cut into small pieces

2 Tbsp apple cider vinegar

1 tsp dijon mustard

2 Tbsp lemon juice, fresh squeezed

1 tsp raw honey

Dash sea salt and pepper

1 cup wild rice, cooked

5 Tbsp olive oil

1/4 cup pistachios

1/4 cup chopped walnuts

1 Tbsp nutritional yeast

In a large salad bowl, combine kale, 2 tablespoons olive oil, salt, and 1 tablespoon of lemon juice. Massage kale until it softens, about 3 minutes. Add the cooked rice, apple, avocado, blueberries, walnuts, and pistachios. To make the dressing, whisk together the remaining olive oil and lemon juice with apple cider vinegar, honey, and mustard. Drizzle over the salad, gently toss, and sprinkle with nutritional yeast. Enjoy right away or pack with you for lunch!

Loaded Lentils

Serves: 4

Vegetarian/vegan meals like this recipe are loaded with nutrients and can last a few days, especially when you're operating a busy schedule. If you're not a lentil or legume fan, cook your protein of choice and use the rest of the recipes to make the dressing and roasted veggies. If you do include grains and legumes in your diet, remember to soak them for 12-24 hours prior to cooking to help with key nutrient absorption. For a non-vegan version, my big splurge when I make this recipe is to add turkey bacon to the turnips and brussels sprouts....and that's all I need to say.

3 medium turnips, diced into 1/2 inch cubes

2 tsp herb seasoning, such as Italian

2 tsp maple syrup

1/3 cup of avocado oil

2 medium sized shallots, finely chopped

2 cups brussels sprouts, thinly sliced

1 cup green lentils

3 cups water

2 Tbsp apple cider vinegar

1/3 cup pumpkin seeds

1/4 cup parsley, finely chopped

salt and pepper to taste

Preheat oven to 425°F and line a baking sheet with parchment paper. In a large bowl, combine the turnips, brussels sprouts, herb seasoning, maple syrup, 3 tablespoons of avocado oil, and a dash of salt. Spread the seasoned turnips and brussels sprouts onto the baking sheet and roast for about 20 minutes until the veggies are cooked through but not too soft. In a large pot, heat 1 tablespoon of avocado oil, add shallots, and cook until softened. Add lentils, cook for a few minutes, then add the water. Bring to a boil, then reduce heat to low and simmer for 30 minutes until the lentils are done. Drain and season with salt to taste. Add the turnips and brussels sprouts to lentils and toss with apple cider vinegar, maple syrup, pumpkin seeds, and parsley. Add additional salt and pepper to taste, and coat with additional avocado oil if needed. Carry on!

Cauli Molly Garlic Soup

Serves: 4

This cauliflower soup will make everyone love the vegetable! It is creamy and provides a great carrier for flavor. Feel free to incorporate your favorite herbal seasoning and even truffle salt to give it a buttery taste. I've used this recipe when I had leftover roasted cauliflower that I had used with another meal. When you're looking for something new or can't think of a different way to present the vegetables, blending them with aromatic herbs and spices is always a great way to combine the flavors.

1 large head cauliflower, cut into chunks

1 yellow onion, diced

1 garlic bulb, top sliced off

3 cups low sodium vegetable broth

3 Tbsp extra virgin olive oil, plus additional for garnish

Dash of cayenne pepper and paprika

Sea salt and pepper to taste

1 Tbsp dried thyme leaves

Preheat oven to 425°F. Place the cauliflower chunks and onion on a baking sheet. Toss evenly with 2 Tbsp of olive oil and season with salt, pepper, cayenne pepper, and paprika. Place the garlic bulb on a piece of foil, drizzle with olive oil, add salt and pepper, and place on the same baking sheet as the cauliflower and onion. Bake for about 40 minutes until cauliflower turns golden brown. Remove the cauliflower and onion from the oven, but keep the garlic roasting. Place the cauliflower and onion in a pot and fill with the vegetable broth. Add the thyme and bring to a boil; season with salt and pepper if needed. Reduce heat to low and simmer for 10 minutes. Ladle the soup into a blender, add the roasted garlic, and blend until smooth. Add nut milk, like cashew milk, if it's too thick. Serve in a bowl and drizzle olive oil over the top. Enjoy on a cool day or anytime!

Collard Veggie Wrap

Serves: 2

What a great way to have your veggies! This wrap is truly filling with its layers of veggies and your protein of choice—veggies or meat. It also makes a great falafel wrap and takes almost anything else you can stuff in it.

Collard greens make for a great wrap, as they are resistant to getting soggy compared to other greens. Make this ahead and pack with you. Have half of it for a snack or eat the whole thing for lunch.

2 collard leaves

10 asparagus spears, roasted and cut in half

1/2 avocado, sliced lengthwise

1 carrot, cut into thin strips

1/2 cucumber, skin peeled off, cut into thin strips

1 cup micro greens

1 cup red cabbage, thinly sliced

4 basil leaves, minced

1/2 cup hummus of choice or cooked chicken breast strips

1/2 cup walnut pieces

Wash and dry the collard leaves. With a paring knife, shave down the stems. You can also blanch the collard greens ahead of time in a pot with hot water to loosen up the fibers in the leaves, then let them cool. Laying the leaves flat, spread 1/4 cup of hummus or cooked chicken breast near the upper/middle part of each leaf, sprinkle with basil, and layer each leaf with asparagus, avocado, carrots, cucumber, micro greens, cabbage, and walnuts. Wrap the leaves as you would wrap a burrito, cut in half and savor the goodness!

Zesty Side Salmon
Serves: 2

This salmon makes for a great main course or a delicious side to any salad or roasted veggies. Pair it with the kale or lentil salad mentioned earlier, or opt for a simple mixed greens concoction. When it comes to seafood, know your source and make sure that the fish is not farm-raised. Most of the time, farm-raised fish has coloring added to it, and the fish is fed things it normally doesn't have in its natural environment. Just as with meat, sustainably sourced is best!

1 lb salmon

1/4 cup olive oil

Salt and pepper

2 Tbsp honey

1 Tbsp minced ginger

1 Tbsp capers

1 Tbsp freshly squeezed lemon juice and 6 thin slices of lemon

2 Tbsp chopped cilantro

3 garlic cloves, minced

Preheat oven to 400°F. Brush salmon with 1 tablespoon of olive oil, and season with salt and pepper. Place salmon on a large piece of foil and fold foil sides to make 1-2 inch wall around the salmon. Place the salmon onto a baking sheet. In a blender, combine the rest of the olive oil, honey, ginger, capers, lemon juice, cilantro, and garlic. Pour the mixture over the salmon to distribute evenly. Layer the lemon slices on top. Bake the salmon uncovered for about 20 minutes. Allow the salmon to cool, then remove from foil. Peel the skin off using a fork, and place salmon on a serving plate. Drizzle with the remaining sauce, and voila!

SATISFYING, END OF THE DAY DINNER RECIPES:

Dinners don't have to be complicated. It's the end of the day, and the last thing you need is a complicated recipe. I always use dinner time as an opportunity to prep for the next day and cook extra to have leftovers. Some of these recipes will call for making your own dressing or sauce, but feel free to substitute with a basic olive oil and apple cider vinegar concoction that you've found in earlier recipes or a sugar cleanse friendly dressing of choice. If you have a little extra time in the evening, this could be a great opportunity to experiment with a new recipe or two. Finding your go-to recipes can be a real treat when you are pushed for time. Keep your essentials (something you frequently cook) in the refrigerator for those nights when you need something quick and healthy. I always have a bunch of vegetables ready to make a stir-fry and lean protein chicken for busy nights. A bonus with most of the dressings is that you can make multiple servings and store in the refrigerator to be used with other meals.

Kale + Pesto + Roasted Veggie Mix

Serves: 2

There are so many ways to enjoy kale. Simply changing the dressing you use and other vegetables you include in the salad can make a huge difference. The roasted carrots and kale combo is one of my favorites. This recipe may look as if it is really involved, but don't let it scare you. I simply broke it down to make prep work easier and your kitchen countertop organized. I recommend making a little extra of the pesto sauce and using it to cook veggies for breakfast or as a marinade.

Roasted Carrots and Chickpeas:

4 large purple carrots

15 oz can chickpeas, drained, rinsed, and dried

2 Tbsp olive oil

Salt and pepper to taste

1 tsp dried parsley

1 tsp dried basil

1/4 tsp garlic powder

Unique Pesto Sauce:

1 bunch, green portion top of carrots

1/4 cup extra virgin olive oil

Salt and pepper to taste

1/2 lemon fresh juice

1/4 cup of almonds or other nut, like cashew or walnut

Salad base:

4 cups kale of choice, thinly sliced, stems removed

1 cup wild rice, cooked

1/2 cup sesame seeds

Preheat oven to 425°F. Line a baking sheet with parchment paper. Cut carrots into rounds about 1/4-inch thick and spread over a baking sheet with the chickpeas. In a bowl, combine the 2 Tbsp olive oil with the rest of the spices, season with salt and pepper to taste, and spread over the carrots and chickpeas to coat evenly. Bake for about 45-50 minutes until carrots are done and chickpeas are crunchy. In a food processor or blender, combine all the ingredients to make the pesto using the high setting. Blend until it forms a smooth paste. In a large salad bowl, mix kale with the pesto until evenly combined, then add the carrots, chickpeas, and wild rice. Top with sesame seeds and serve as a side or a main course!

Pho Sure So Good

Serves: 2

This is one of my favorite recipes to recommend for when you need something cleansing, you're craving a soup, or you're looking for a simple, all-in-one nourishing meal. Share with a friend, or have it all to yourself! The zucchini and beef absorb the flavors even more given another day, so make a little extra and savor it the next day. I always like to offer vegan or vegetarian options—instead of beef, you can have tempeh or tofu. I would recommend baking the tofu for 20-30 minutes with olive oil and the spices listed before adding it to the soup to lock in the flavor and give it some texture. Remember, make the recipe your own!

1 yellow onion, diced

1 Tbsp of minced ginger

1/4 tsp cinnamon powder

3 whole cloves

3 garlic cloves, minced

3 Tbsp olive oil

2 Tbsp fish sauce

32 oz beef broth or bone broth of choice

1/2 package kelp noodles or rice noodles

1 medium zucchini, chopped or spiralized

1/2 lbs beef, thinly sliced

Salt and pepper to taste

Bean sprouts, basil, cilantro, and lime to taste

In a large saucepan, heat the olive oil. Stir in the onion, garlic, and spices, including ginger, and cook for a few minutes until the onion becomes translucent. Add the zucchini and cook for another couple of minutes. Season beef with salt and pepper and add it to the saucepan. When the beef is browned evenly on both sides, pour in the broth and fish sauce and bring to a gentle simmer. Add the noodles and cook for 15 minutes, depending on which noodles you use. Serve in two bowls and top with bean sprouts, basil, cilantro, and lime. Season to taste with salt and pepper...and enjoy the warmth and nutrition of the broth!

Sweet and Spicy Sweet Potato, Broccoli "Rice" Salad

Serves: 6

If you are doing the 14-day sugar cleanse, this is not the recipe to use, as it has sweet potatoes and raisins. However, this is an excellent recipe for when you've rewired your taste buds, have completed the cleanse, and are ready to get back to a healthier and more satisfying way of eating. The only reason root vegetables are not part of the cleanse (even though they are nutritionally dense) is because of the starch content. This is one of my favorite meals for a main course, a side dish, or even a snack. When I was taming my sweet tooth, the sweet potatoes were an excellent carbohydrate source, as they were satisfying and filling and provided just enough sweetness to get rid of the sugar monster within.

Salad:

2 large sweet potatoes, peeled and cut into 1/2 inch cubes

2 Tbsp coconut oil or ghee, melted

4 cups cauliflower cut into bite size pieces

1/4 tsp garlic salt to taste

1/2 cup Italian parsley, finely chopped

1/4 cup slivered almonds

1/4 cup raisins

1/4 cup hemp seeds

Dressing:

1/4 cup coconut oil, melted

1/4 cup almond butter

1 Tbsp apple cider vinegar

1 tsp honey or maple syrup

1 tsp curry powder

2 tsp Sriracha sauce

pinch of salt

Preheat oven to 425°F. Line a baking sheet with parchment paper. Place the cubed sweet potatoes onto the baking sheet, drizzle with 1 Tbsp of coconut oil, coat evenly, and place in the oven. Bake for approximately 20-30 minutes until they are done.

Place broccoli in a food processor on high setting until it breaks down into small, rice size pieces. In a large pan, heat 1 Tbsp of coconut oil and stir in the broccoli. Cook for about 5 minutes, stirring occasionally until the broccoli is golden brown. Sprinkle with garlic salt. In a medium bowl, combine the dressing ingredients, adjusting the spice of Sriracha sauce to taste. Place the cauliflower and sweet potatoes into a large bowl, cover with raisins, slivered almonds, hemp seeds, and Italian parsley. Pour in the dressing and mix gently into the salad. Season with salt if needed. Kick back and relax!

Portobello Cap Salad with Cashew Strawberry Dressing

Serves: 2

One reason I love portobello mushrooms is because of their texture and flavor.

They have a meaty texture that's great when you're trying to have a vegetarian meal but still want something hearty that will carry flavor nicely. This salad is super refreshing with the strawberries and lemon, and provides plenty of healthy fats and natural sweetness to keep you satisfied!

1 cup wild rice, cooked

2 portobello caps, save stems for a future soup

1/4 cup plus 1 Tbsp extra virgin olive oil

1 Tbsp parsley, finely chopped

1 1/2 cups radicchio, shredded

3 cups of arugula

1/4 cup walnut pieces

1/2 cup strawberries

1/4 cup cashews

1 Tbsp lemon

2 tsp maple syrup

Salt to taste

Preheat oven to 400°F. Brush the portobello caps with 1 Tbsp of olive oil, and evenly distribute the parsley along with a little salt. Prepare a baking sheet and place the caps gill side down. Bake for 15 minutes. In a blender, combine the strawberries, cashews, lemon, and maple syrup to make the dressing. In a salad bowl, combine the arugula, wild rice, radicchio, and walnut pieces. Drizzle with the strawberry dressing, and season with salt to taste. Plate the salad and place sliced portobello caps on top of the salad. You may have some dressing leftover, and if not, it's easy to make more!

Curry Quinoa—The Slow Cooker Way

Serves: 6-8 serving

Talk about a flavor packed meal waiting for you when you come home at the end of the day! It's meals like these that make eating healthy so simple and delicious. The slower cooker can truly be a life saver for those times when you need meals for multiple days, you've got lots of mouths to feed, or you want to keep dinners and next-day lunches simple, but nutritious. If you're doing the 14-day cleanse, you can substitute turnips, brussels sprouts, or cauliflower for the squash. Enjoy this meal any time, as it makes great leftovers.

1 medium butternut squash, peeled and cubed

1 large broccoli head, cut into small florets

1/2 yellow onion, diced

1 can organic chickpeas, drained

3 cups vegetable broth

2 cans coconut milk

1/4 cup quinoa

1 Tbsp ginger, grated

2 tsp turmeric powder

2 tsp curry powder

1 tsp of coconut aminos

1/2 tsp salt

Add all ingredients to the slow cooker and stir gently to combine. Cook for approximately 3-4 hours on low setting. Periodically, check the squash to see if it's done, as cooking times may vary. Some toppings to consider include cilantro, chives, or homemade roasted pumpkin seeds!

For more recipe and meal ideas and ways to supercharge your health, follow me on:

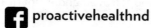 proactivehealthnd

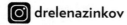 drelenazinkov

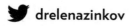 drelenazinkov

Acknowledgements

Writing this book would not have been possible without the unwavering support, humor, and love of my husband. Thank you, Stanislav, for being my rock, for knowing when it's time for a little laughter, and for being the greatest partner I could have on this incredible journey. To my son, Slava, thank you for challenging my perception of what's possible when you only have a few minutes in a day.

I'd like to thank my colleagues, the professors at Bastyr University, and my patients, all of whom have contributed to my growth and understanding of the human body—I continue to strive to be a better doctor each and every day, and I am grateful to be part of medicine that focuses on treating people rather than symptoms.

I am grateful to my editor Arielle Eckstut and my team at JKS Communications for their incredible knowledge and support, and for helping me get my message to the world.

Bibliography

1. Wurtman, R. J., and Wurtman, J. J. (1995). "Brain Serotonin, Carbohydrate-Craving, Obesity and Depression." *Obesity Research*, 3(S4). doi:10.1002/j.1550-8528.1995.tb00215.x

2. Anderson, R. A. (2008). "Chromium and polyphenols from cinnamon improve insulin sensitivity." *Proceedings of the Nutrition Society*, 67(01), 48-53. doi:10.1017/s0029665108006010

3. Ranganathan, V. K.; Siemionow, V.; Liu, J. Z.; Sahgal, V.; and Yue, G. H. (2004). "From mental power to muscle power—gaining strength by using the mind." *Neuropsychologia*, 42(7), 944-956. doi:10.1016/j.neuropsychologia.2003.11.018

4. Talbot, M., and McTaggart, L. (2011). *The Holographic Universe: The Revolutionary Theory of Reality*. New York, NY: Harper Perennial.

5. "How Intermittent Movement Benefits Your Health." *Mercola.com*, fitness.mercola.com/sites/fitness/archive/2014/04/11/intermittent-movement.aspx.

6. King, J. A.; Wasse, L. K.; Stensel, D. J.; and Nimmo, M. A. (2013). "Exercise and ghrelin. A narrative overview of research." *Appetite*, 68, 83-91. doi:10.1016/j.appet.2013.04.018

7. Zheng, X., and Niu, S. (2018). "Leptin-induced basal Akt phosphorylation and its implication in exercise-mediated improvement of

insulin sensitivity. *Biochemical and Biophysical Research Communications, 496*(1), 37-43. doi:10.1016/j.bbrc.2017.12.161

8. Maskell, James. *The Evolution of Medicine: Join the Movement to Solve Chronic Disease and Fall Back in Love with Medicine* (Kindle Locations 387-389). Knew Publishing. Kindle Edition.

9. "How to Rewire Your Brain to End Food Cravings." (2013, February 21). Retrieved October 27, 2017, from http://drhyman.com/blog/2012/07/16/how-to-rewire-your-brain-to-end-food-cravings-2/

10. Ukkola, O., and Santaniemi, M. (2002). "Adiponectin: a link between excess adiposity and associated comorbidities?" *Journal of Molecular Medicine, 80*(11), 696-702. doi:10.1007/s00109-002-0378-7

11. Levy, E., Ménard, D., Delvin, E., Stan, S., Mitchell, G., Lambert, M., . . . Seidman, E. (2001). "The Polymorphism at Codon 54 of the FABP2 Gene Increases Fat Absorption in Human Intestinal Explants." *Journal of Biological Chemistry, 276*(43), 39679-39684. doi:10.1074/jbc.m105713200

12. Thumser, Alfred E.; Moore, Jennifer Bernadette; Plant, Nick J. *Current Opinion in Clinical Nutrition and Metabolic Care.* (March 2014). Volume 17, Issue 2, p 124–129.

13. *Nature Reviews Neuroscience* 12, 453-466 (August 2011) | doi:10.1038/nrn3071

14. World J "Gastroenterol." 2015 Aug 7; 21(29): 8787–8803. Published online 2015 Aug 7. doi: 10.3748/wjg.v21.i29.8787

15. Conlon, M. A., and Bird, A. R. (2014, December 24). "The Impact of Diet and Lifestyle on Gut Microbiota and Human Health." Retrieved February 19, 2018, from http://www.mdpi.com/2072-6643/7/1/1716.

16. *Bioessays.* 2014 Oct; 36(10): 940–949.Published online 2014 Aug 8. doi: 10.1002/bies.201400071

17. Colberg, P. S. (n.d.). "Increasing Insulin Sensitivity." Retrieved February 20, 2018, from https://www.diabetesselfmanagement.com/managing-diabetes/treatment-approaches/increasing-insulin-sensitivity/

18. Marliss, E. B., and Vranic, M. (2002, February 01). "Intense Exercise Has Unique Effects on Both Insulin Release and Its Roles in Glucoregulation." Retrieved February 20, 2018, from http://diabetes.diabetesjournals.org/content/51/suppl_1/S271

19. Kirsten Weir. December 2011, Vol 42, No. 11. American Psychological Association. Print version: page 48 http://www.apa.org/monitor/2011/12/exercise.aspx

20. McGonigal, K. (2011, November 27). "How Mindfulness Makes the Brain Immune to Temptation." Retrieved February 19, 2018, from https://www.psychologytoday.com/blog/the-science-willpower/201111/how-mindfulness-makes-the-brain-immune-temptation

21. "What Eating Nothing But McDonalds for 10 Days Does to Gut Bacteria." (n.d.). Retrieved February 19, 2018, from http://time.com/3853618/mcdonalds-gut-bacteria/

22. Myles, I. A. (2014, June 17). "Fast food fever: reviewing the impacts of the Western diet on immunity." Retrieved February 19, 2018, from https://www.ncbi.nlm.nih.gov/pubmed/24939238

23. Sabater-Molina, M.; Larqué, E.; Torrella, F.; and Zamora, S. (2009, September). "Dietary fructooligosaccharides and potential benefits on health." Retrieved February 19, 2018, from https://www.ncbi.nlm.nih.gov/pubmed/20119826

24. (2018, February 12). "Seven Foods to Supercharge Your Gut Bacteria." Retrieved February 19, 2018, from http://www.pcrm.org/media/online/sept2014/seven-foods-to-supercharge-your-gut-bacteria

25. "Glutamine and the preservation of gut integrity." R.R.W.J. van der Hulst, MD; M.F. von Meyenfeldt, MD; N.E.P. Deutz, MD; P.B. Soeters, MD (Prof); R.J.M. Brummer, MD; B.K. von Kreel; PhD, J.W. Arends, MD (Prof) Published: 29 May 1993

26. Costello, R.; Wallace, T. C.; and Rosanoff, A. (2016, January 07). "Magnesium | Advances in Nutrition | Oxford Academic." Retrieved February 19, 2018, from http://advances.nutrition.org/content/7/1/199.full

27. Hemarajata, P., and Versalovic, J. (2012). "Effects of probiotics on gut microbiota: mechanisms of intestinal immunomodulation and neuromodulation." *Therapeutic Advances in Gastroenterology*, 6(1), 39-51. doi:10.1177/1756283x12459294

28. Bischoff, S. C. (2011, March 14). "'Gut health': a new objective in medicine?" Retrieved February 19, 2018, from https://bmcmedicine.biomedcentral.com/articles/10.1186/1741-7015-9-24

29. "Licorice. Evid Based Complement Alternat Med." 2012; 2012: 216970. Published online 2011 Jun 16.

30. Mora-Rodriguez, R., and Coyle, E. F. (2000). "Effects of plasma epinephrine on fat metabolism during exercise: interactions with exercise intensity." *American Journal of Physiology-Endocrinology and Metabolism, 278*(4). doi:10.1152/ajpendo.2000.278.4.e669

31. "Food Cravings - What do they Mean?" Colleen Huber, NMD. (n.d.). Retrieved February 19, 2018, from https://natureworksbest. com/naturopathy-works/food-cravings/

32. Pick, M. (2013). *"Is it me or my adrenals?: Your proven 30-day program for overcoming adrenal fatigue and feeling fantastic again."* Carlsbad, CA: Hay House.

33. Gómez-Pinilla, F. (2008, July 01). "Brain foods: the effects of nutrients on brain function." Retrieved February 19, 2018, from https:// www.nature.com/articles/nrn2421

34. "In this office, desks are for working, not eating lunch." (2017, June 01). Retrieved February 20, 2018, from https://www.theglobeandmail.com/report-on-business/industry-news/property-report/in-this-office-desks-are-for-working-not-eating-lunch/article34153148/

35. Grossman, P.; Niemann, L.; Schmidt, S.; and Walach, H. (2004, July). "Mindfulness-based stress reduction and health benefits. A meta-analysis." Retrieved February 19, 2018, from https://www. ncbi.nlm.nih.gov/pubmed/15256293

36. Bloom, H. (2000). *Global Brain: the Evolution of Mass Mind from the Big Bang to the 21st Century.* New York: John Wiley & Sons.

37. Leeds, U. O. (2009, December 16). "Sheep in human clothing - scientists reveal our flock mentality." Retrieved February 19, 2018, from http://www.leeds.ac.uk/news/article/397/sheep_in_human_ clothing__scientists_reveal_our_flock_mentality

38. Warren, R.; Amen, D. G.; and Hyman, M. (2013). *The Daniel Plan: 40 days to a Healthier Life.* Grand Rapids, MI: Harpercollins Christian Pub.

39. (n.d.). "Stress Hormone Receptors Localized in Sweet Taste Cells." Retrieved February 19, 2018, from http://www.monell.org/news/ news_releases/

40. Wansink, B. (2004). "Environmental Factors That Increase the Food Intake and Consumption Volume of Unknowing Consumers." *Annual Review of Nutrition, 24*(1), 455-479. doi:10.1146/annurev. nutr.24.012003.132140

41. Shoham, N.; Girshovitz, P.; Katzengold, R.; Shaked, N.; Benayahu, D.; and Gefen, A. (2014). "Adipocyte Stiffness Increases with Accumulation of Lipid Droplets." *Biophysical Journal, 106*(6), 1421-1431. doi:10.1016/j.bpj.2014.01.045

42. Wise, R. A. (1998). "Drug-activation of brain reward pathways." *Drug and Alcohol Dependence, 51*(1-2), 13-22. doi:10.1016/s0376-8716(98)00063-5

43. Publishing, H. H. (n.d.). "Overcoming Addiction: Find an effective path toward recovery." Retrieved February 19, 2018, from https://www.health.harvard.edu/special-health-reports/overcoming-addiction-paths-toward-recovery

44. Avena, N. M.; Rada, P.; and Hoebel, B. G. (2008). "Evidence for sugar addiction: Behavioral and neurochemical effects of intermittent, excessive sugar intake." *Neuroscience & Biobehavioral Reviews, 32*(1), 20-39. doi:10.1016/j.neubiorev.2007.04.019

45. Thompson, D. (2014, September 17). "A Formula for Perfect Productivity: Work for 52 Minutes, Break for 17." Retrieved February 20, 2018, from https://www.theatlantic.com/business/archive/2014/09/science-tells-you-how-many-minutes-should-you-take-a-break-for-work-17/380369/

46. Shi, D.; Nikodijević, O.; Jacobson, K. A.; and Daly, J. W. (1993). "Chronic caffeine alters the density of adenosine, adrenergic, cholinergic, GABA, and serotonin receptors and calcium channels in mouse brain." *Cellular and Molecular Neurobiology, 13*(3), 247-261. doi:10.1007/bf00733753

47. Wurtman, J. J., and Frusztajer, N. T. (2010). *The Serotonin Power Diet*. Emmaus, PA: Rodale.

48. Drewnowski, A. (1997). "Nontasters, Tasters, and Supertasters of 6-n-Propylthiouracil (PROP) and Hedonic Response to Sweet." *Physiology and Behavior, 62*(3), 649-655. doi:10.1016/s0031-9384(97)00193-5

49. Tepper, B. J. (1998). "6-n-Propylthiouracil: A Genetic Marker for Taste, with Implications for Food Preference and Dietary Habits." *The American Journal of Human Genetics, 63*(5), 1271-1276. doi:10.1086/302124

50. Stice, E.; Yokum, S.; Zald, D.; and Dagher, A. (2010). "Dopamine-Based Reward Circuitry Responsivity, Genetics, and Overeating." *Behavioral Neurobiology of Eating Disorders Current Topics in Behavioral Neurosciences*, 81-93. doi 10.1007/7854_2010_89

51. Stice, E.; Yokum, S.; Bohon, C.; Marti, N.; and Smolen, A. (2010). "Reward circuitry responsivity to food predicts future increases in body mass: Moderating effects of DRD2 and DRD4." *NeuroImage*, *50*(4), 1618-1625. doi:10.1016/j.neuroimage.2010.01.081

52. "The Craving Brain." (2014, February 11). Retrieved February 20, 2018, from http://now.tufts.edu/articles/craving-brain

53. Baksa, P. (2011). *The Point of Power*. Ashland, OH: Intelegance.

Index